94807

D0225442

Childbirth in the Global Village

Is the experience of childbirth becoming 'globalised'?
Is the encroachment of the western medical model
dehumanising a profoundly human experience?
If so, what can midwives and midwife educators
do about it?

These are the questions at the heart of *Childbirth in the Global Village* which highlights the role that globalisation plays in changing childbirth practices and its implications for midwifery practice and education.

Built around the vivid personal stories of women and midwives experiencing childbirth in four very different cultures – Africa, Malaysia, North America and England – the book reveals the interactions between the powerful messages of the media, the dominance of medical/scientific 'knowledge' and the role played by global institutions and the academy.

Childbirth in the Global Village will resonate with the experience of midwives everywhere and makes a strong case for redesigning the midwifery curriculum to reflect the interconnectedness of childbirth, midwifery education and practice around the globe.

Dawn Hillier is an experienced midwife and Dean of the School of Health Care Practice at Anglia Polytechnic University.

Childbirth in the Global Village

Implications for Midwifery Education and Practice

Dawn Hillier

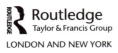
Routledge
Taylor & Francis Group

LONDON AND NEW YORK

First published 2003
by Routledge
11 New Fetter Lane, London EC4P 4EE

Simultaneously published in the USA and Canada
by Routledge
29 West 35th Street, New York, NY 10001

Routledge is an imprint of the Taylor & Francis Group

© 2003 Dawn Hillier

Typeset in Times by RefineCatch Limited, Bungay, Suffolk
Printed and bound in Great Britain by
Biddles Ltd, Guildford & King's Lynn

British Library Cataloguing in Publication Data
A catalogue record for this book is available from the British Library

Library of Congress Cataloging in Publication Data
Hillier, Dawn, 1950–
    Childbirth in the global village : implications for midwifery
education and practice / Dawn Hillier
        p. cm.
    Includes bibliographical references and index.
    ISBN 0–415–27551–2 – ISBN 0–415–27552–0 (pbk.)
    1. Childbirth – Cross-cultural studies. 2. Globalization – Health
aspects. 3. Midwives – Education. 4. Obstetrics – Social aspects.
I. Title.
    RG950.H54 2003
    618.2 – dc21   2002037169

ISBN 0–415–27551–2 HB
ISBN 0–415–27552–0 PB

Contents

List of figures

Acknowledgements

This book would not have been possible without the contributions and help of a large number of people. I would first like to thank Professor Peter Jarvis who has been my guide and friend for many years. His encouragement and support, his endless enthusiasm and intellectual rigour have been an inspiration.

My gratitude and thanks must next go to my colleagues at work who have supported and encouraged, commiserated with and cajoled me along the way. I am indebted to the Sir Winston Churchill Travelling Fellowship for triggering the research that underpins this book and for providing the financial resources for my fieldtrip to Africa.

My deepest appreciation goes particularly to the women I encountered throughout my travels around the world who taught me their ways of birth and what it means to be a midwife. The midwives, nurses, doctors and health officials who have facilitated my work are too numerous to mention by name, and so I thank them collectively.

Finally, I want to express my special thanks to my family who have borne the burden of an absent mother and wife, sister and aunt over several years while I immersed myself in my study. To John, my husband, goes my deepest gratitude for his patience, understanding and support.

Preface

The concept of the new world order was first derived from a United Nations resolution (1974) proclaiming a determination to work for, among other things, common interests, interdependence, and cooperation between nations. This aimed to eliminate gaps between 'developed and developing' countries; to ensure accelerated economic and social development; to correct inequalities and redress existing injustices thereby ensuring peace and justice for present and future generations. All this is based on the premise that an international distribution of knowledge is an essential prerequisite for these far-reaching objectives and it is this premise that draws midwifery education and its role in the preservation of maternal and child health into the framework of development.

The role and status of global institutions and researchers in the process of disseminating knowledge and in the exercise of economic power are, however, linked with the fact that modern science and technology are largely the products of industrialised nations. Western scientific knowledge, however, is not only problematic to those at the outer edges who feel the effects of globalisation slightly later, but is also problematical for women and midwives in the West under the conditions of postmodernity.

This book is concerned with the impact of the new world order on women's experience of childbirth illustrated through the stories of women in Africa, Malaysia, America and England.

Chapter 1

Women's stories, women's lives

Four women's stories

Ama's story

Ama gently woke me. Whispering so as not to disturb the other occupants of the hut, she pantomimed gestures to ensure my understanding. Victoria, my guide and translator, had spent the night with another family in the village.

It was still dark outside. It was also surprisingly cold, but I knew it would become very hot once the sun was up. Ama lit an oil lamp – there was no electricity – and started a fire to prepare some food.

While the porridge was cooking, she bathed herself and the children, using water she had collected the evening before. The children were thin with large abdomens but they smiled and giggled as she told them a story, which Victoria had arrived in time to translate.

Ama handed me a brightly coloured plastic bowl with what looked like gruel in it. She looked apologetic and sad. It was not much and she gave herself even less. After breakfast, Ama's nine-year-old son, who had a long walk to school, set off. It was just after 5 a.m.

We left Victoria behind and set off for the fields. Ama was carrying her nine-month-old baby on her back. In one hand she had a hoe. Over the other arm she carried food and water wrapped in a bundle. Her young daughter followed behind with a large tin can on her head. She was about five years old. Girls learn domestic chores and help in the home from a very early age.

Ama was heavily pregnant and she bent almost double all day as she tilled the soil. She had provided me with a hoe so that I could help, but I did not have her stamina and had to frequently retreat to a nearby tree to rest. It was very hot and the work repetitive and hard. The soil was dry and dusty and clogged my eyes, nose and mouth. By the end of the day the red dust had penetrated my clothing down to my underwear.

At sunset, Ama, her children and I made our way home. We collected water in the large tin can and firewood, which she and her daughter carried on their heads. Balancing a bundle of firewood on my head was a skill acquired over the three-mile walk back to the village along the dusty track. Despite our tiredness, Ama attempted to teach me to carry the water can on my head which afforded them both a great deal of amusement.

When we reached the hut, Ama settled the baby on the ground, then began to prepare the main meal of the day. She announced that we would have a special meal – lye soup and fufu. I suspected this was a reward for my hard work.

Ama lit a fire outside her hut. The other women were doing the same. There was a general air of camaraderie among the women. Calling out to each other, sharing their day and telling stories. Victoria could not translate fast enough and there was a great deal of joking and laughter. I could not understand what was being said but I understood the feelings being expressed through their gestures and generosity.

Victoria informed me that it was a great honour to be given chicken since the villagers rarely eat meat but she said they would be offended if I refused to eat the meal. For some reason Ama seemed revived with the thought of preparing a special treat for her guests and family. The other women began to arrive with gifts of food too. Some rice, yams, plantains and oranges. It would be a feast. The village elders came to join in the gathering and began to ask questions about my life in England. The children gathered around to listen. Visitors were rare and a great source of entertainment.

The sound of hollow, regular drumming was carried on the evening breeze. The women were pounding fufu, the staple food of these Ghanaians that usually accompanies soup.

After the meal the women started to dance and sing. They had dressed in different clothes and put on their beads. They were clearly in a mood to celebrate. It was dark and the only light came from the campfires and oil lamps. Victoria informed me that as with the symbolic designs on the clothes worn by the women, each dance movement conveyed a recognisable message and meaning. For Ghanaians, dance is a dramatic expression of life itself as important as language and conveys a whole range of experiences. Drumming and singing are essential accompaniments to dance, setting the scene and creating the mood. The dancing sometimes follows the music but it can be in opposition to it for dramatic effect.

After the small celebration, Ama and the other women cleared up and then gathered what yam and plantain they could spare to take to the local town. We began the long walk along the dark road into the nearest town, which was about six miles away. On arrival Ama and the other women set up roadside kitchens. They fried yam and sold it to passers by. The income would supplement their diet and provide needed cash for school fees, clothes, and other things for the children.

Ama and her friends returned home to await the return of their husbands from the local bar where they had been drinking fermented palm wine. Ama had to attend to her husband's needs before she could retire for the night. Soon it was time to rise again. Ama was tired. I sympathised with her. I was tired too but I was leaving that day. Ama's life would continue, long after I had gone, along its traditional path.

(Ama, Ghana, 1991)

Emefa's story

In another village, Emefa is about to give birth to her fourth child. Huddled in a corner of the hut she was lying on the floor, or rather on a piece of thin cloth that was once brightly coloured. No cushion or comfort as we would know it. No pillow for her head and no mattress for her back. She lay curled into a small ball on her left side, her pregnant and contracting uterus protruding from her thin frame. No sound came from her. No sound came from the midwife either. She was seated in the corner of the dark hot hut, waiting. Suddenly, Emefa gave a low whimper and hauled herself into a sitting and then squatting position. The midwife crept over to her and gently supported Emefa's back as she bore down. No words, no commands, no yelling. The expulsive contraction was handled in a quiet and dignified fashion. Once it was over, Emefa lay down on the ground again to rest until she was required to continue the process of giving birth. Her body was practised in the art of birthing. She had already had three children before. Another contraction gripped Emefa and she lumbered up into her squatting position again. This time, the midwife crouched in front of her, waiting. The baby's head appeared gradually, slowly making its progress into the world. How did the midwife know that it was time? No words had been spoken by either of them. It was almost mystical. A kind of unseen and unheard language passed between Emefa and the midwife. It was as if Emefa's body had communicated its readiness to the midwife and she needed no verbal information to guide her in what was happening to Emefa at that precise moment in time. A soft whoosh and the baby's body was born into the steady and confident hands of the midwife. And still there was no sound. The baby did not cry, not because there was any problem, but because it was a gentle birth. The baby was breathing and at once handed to his mother – a boy at last. She had had three girls before. Her husband would be pleased and the village would rejoice.

(Emefa, Ghana, 1991)

Six weeks later I was visiting a small village in Malawi where I met another woman during childbirth. Sitting in the shade of nearby trees, a group of women were making the traditional porridge given to labouring women to provide energy for the hard work ahead. These women were the friends and relatives of the labouring woman and they were there to assist the midwife and give support – a show of solidarity in their womanhood. As they stirred the gruel, they chatted about the family, the strife, the joys and events that shaped their lives. Any conflict was resolved during these meetings since conflict could delay the birth and cause complications. The women's chatter was interspersed with songs and stories of bygone days and important events in the community. The elders told of the line of descent and ancestry of the new baby, creating his or her identity and place within the life of the village. In a hut close by, the labouring woman was nearing her time. The midwife moved between the hut and the group of women, listening. She knew the family; knew their history and physical condition. She had delivered the young woman herself with the help of her husband. Indeed, she had delivered the young woman's own mother as well. She did not anticipate any problems. The labouring woman was healthy and well nourished. She had no reason to be concerned. She went about the business of preparing for the birth. The women took turns in visiting the labouring woman in the hut to offer encouragement, to massage her or feed her some of the porridge or just sit silently in the corner offering a reassuring presence. This was the young woman's first child. Everyone was looking forward to a new member of the family, especially if it was a girl.

I had sat throughout the whole experience neither speaking nor moving. I had a strong feeling that I must not distract the woman or intrude upon her birth in any way. She was in control. The midwife was there to support and tend to her needs, not to interfere with the process. She neither examined nor issued instructions to the woman. Nature was allowed to take its course and the woman's body was trusted to perform as it was meant to. Later I asked the midwife how she knew that the birth was imminent. She said she just knew. The way in which the woman moved and breathed let her know.

A few years later in Kuala Lumpur, Malaysia, I encountered a woman who was lying in a crowded corridor, clinging to the rails of her trolley and crying out in pain. People were walking by on all sides but none came to her aid. My translator told me that she was saying that the baby was coming. But no one was taking any notice. I placed my hand on her arm to offer some comfort and asked my guide why the woman was in the busy thoroughfare.

'There are no delivery beds available and she is a third class patient in any case. Privacy is not an option for her.' The woman was alone. There was no room for family attendants. Eventually someone came to assist the woman and called the doctors and nurses who were swarming about in their theatre gowns, wearing masks and gloves among the general chaos of the corridor with other people wandering all around. Not even screens were available as the woman began to deliver her baby in the middle of the corridor. This was the best the hospital could offer in the circumstances. One hundred per cent hospital confinement is insisted upon and doctors delivered the babies. In a city that was populated by more than 1,145,342 (1996), state provision for health services was stretched to the limits.

As the baby slid out of his mother, he was limp, blue and covered with a green slime. He was not breathing. The nurse grabbed him and rushed off to find help to resuscitate him. In the panic, no one told the mother what was happening and she screamed in terror. The doctor was called away to another patient and the woman was left alone. The placenta had not yet been delivered.

On the next floor in the private patients' wing, a woman was labouring in a comfortable room with all the technical equipment available in case of an emergency. She had her husband with her. Clearly middle-class, the woman had requested the presence of two of her female relatives, which was granted. A nurse was also present throughout. As the baby began to make her appearance into the world, the doctor was called to conduct the delivery. He had been called away from the woman in the corridor.

Lisa's story

On the other side of the world in Williamsport, Pennsylvania, USA, Lisa prepared to give birth. Lisa graduated in 1985 from a college in New York with a degree in biology and planned to pursue a career in medical research. But Lisa had always loved to act and she joined a small theatre company playing to schools. Later she joined an improvisational team and started to land small parts in television shows. Lisa married at the age of twenty-five and recently celebrated her thirty-ninth birthday. In this account she is looking forward to the birth of her first child.

My estimated due date came and went with no signs that I was anywhere near ready to give birth. My cervix had not ripened and I wasn't dilated at all. The midwife suggested prostaglandin gel applications the following Monday if I hadn't made any progress by then. To cut a long story short, I had three prostaglandin gel applications on the following Monday and Tuesday. The gel was successful in ripening my cervix, but it did not bring on labour and I was only one 'fingertip' dilated. The midwife, after consulting with a doctor, wanted to induce labour the following week. Since it was a holiday weekend and their office would be closed for three days, I was going to have to go to the hospital over the weekend so the baby could be monitored.

Luckily, the following Friday my waters broke at around 12.45 a.m. after going to the bathroom. I had been having some mild contractions while I was watching television that night but didn't think anything of it. My waters were meconium stained, so I called the midwife. She instructed me to get to the hospital right away.

By the time we were on the way to the hospital, the contractions were coming about every 5 minutes but weren't too strong then. When I got to the hospital, they hooked me up to the monitor for close to an hour to monitor the baby. The baby was fine. So, I started to walk about and rock in the chair during the early stages of labour. It didn't take long for the contractions to become stronger. They were 3 to 5 minutes apart and were pretty intense, or so I thought. The nurse told me that they were nothing compared to what I was in for. I tried to use the breathing techniques I learned in our childbirth class, but they weren't working very well. The contractions were close together and steadily building in intensity.

Around 5 a.m. one of the doctors from my midwife's group came in to examine me to see how far along I was since my midwife hadn't arrived at the hospital yet. She said that I was 4 centimetres and 90 per cent effaced. By that time, I was in pain. The contractions were about every 3 minutes and were very strong. The midwife had told the nurses to tell me that I could either go in the tub or have a pain-relieving drug. I didn't want to leave the room so I opted for the injection. After that I was able to rest between contractions.

The midwife arrived and so did my mother, father, sister and sister-in-law. They were all in the room with me while I was in labour. The midwife examined me and announced that I was around 8 centimetres dilated. Around 8.45 a.m. or so, I started to get the urge to push. The midwife examined me and said that I was 9 centimetres dilated. She did not, however, discourage me from pushing. In fact, she encouraged me to push when I felt the urge. I stayed at 9 centimetres for only a short period of time. When she examined me again, she said there was still a little lip on the cervix so she wanted me to push through the next couple of contractions, which I did. All through this pushing, I was not in the position of giving birth. She just encouraged me to push lying on my side.

Around 9.30 a.m. the midwife encouraged me to sit up so that I could start pushing in earnest. After only twenty minutes of pushing, my baby daughter was born. It was the most amazing feeling. Even though I had had an injection I was wide awake and aware of everything that was going on. I saw her head being born, followed by the rest of her body. The midwife put her on my stomach very briefly because she had to be examined immediately by a neonatologist because my waters had been meconium stained. She hadn't swallowed any meconium and was very healthy. She weighed a healthy 7 pounds 8 ounces and she had a full head of black hair.

(Lisa, Pennsylvania, 1995)

Melody's story

Meanwhile, in England, Melody, pregnant for the second time, had planned to have a domino delivery in which her community midwife would deliver her baby in hospital and she and the baby would return home six hours later. All through the pregnancy Melody had seen her community midwife, Sara, and she was confident that all would go smoothly. Sara had delivered Melody's first child two years previously and knew the family well. Melody had given up work as a part-time teacher at the end of summer term and now was enjoying the warm weather and playing with her son, James, in the garden of their small house at the edge of town.

In the early hours of Wednesday morning, Melody woke as her 'waters' had broken. She was not having any contractions as yet but as her previous labour had been quite short she thought she had better contact Sara. After waking her partner, Melody rang her mother and sister who were going to look after James while Melody was giving birth. Sara arrived just as the contractions began to increase and she stayed with Melody for the next hour as the contractions grew stronger and more frequent. Soon afterward Sara suggested that Melody and her partner should make their way to the hospital.

At the hospital, Sara undertook the usual admission procedures; the half-hour fetal heart monitoring that was required by hospital policy, the vaginal examination and the commencement of the partogram. Skipping the ritual bath, Sara encouraged Melody to put on one of her own nightdresses and lie on the bed. By now the contractions were very frequent and Melody was experiencing some urges to push. Sara, an advocate of gentle birth, darkened the room and turned on the music Melody had chosen during her pregnancy. Sara encouraged Melody to lie on her side and suggested that her partner massage the lower part of her back during contractions. Soon the urge to push was overwhelming, Melody gave a grunt, and the baby's head emerged gently and smoothly followed by the baby's body. A lusty cry followed and the baby was immediately put into her mother's arms and Melody put her to the breast. Melody's partner cut the cord and mother and baby were covered with a soft blanket to keep them warm. Twenty minutes later, the placenta delivered, observations of vital signs made, records completed, the mother and baby settled down for a few hours' sleep before returning home to be cared for by Melody's mother, sister and the midwife who would visit regularly for the next ten days.

(Melody, England, 1999)

Cultural messages

According to Davis-Floyd (1992: 44) the rituals of initiatory rites of passage convey symbolic messages that speak of a culture's most deeply held values and beliefs. Many of today's modern societies' deeply held beliefs and values derive from the model of reality inherited from the scientific and industrial revolution in Europe. The machine became the underlying metaphor for the organisation of human life during the seventeenth century with the rapid commercial expansion of Western society (Merchant, 1983). Descartes, Bacon and Hobbs, among others, developed and widely disseminated a philosophy that assumed the universe was mechanistic, following predictable laws rather than the previously held view of the universe as being a living organism infused with a female 'world-soul'. Those who freed themselves from the limited medieval superstitions of the past could discover the universe through science and, moreover, could manipulate it through technology. Within the framework of these philosophies, according to Merchant (ibid.: 193), nature, society and the human body soon became interchangeable fragments that could, legitimately, be replaced or manipulated by external rather than inherent forces.

In a world that is increasingly global, with increased migration and communication systems, all societies and cultures are becoming increasingly pluralistic. Moreover, the distance between cultures is diminishing as we experience what Giddens (1991) terms time-space distanciation, or in Harvey's terms time-space compression (1989). At the same time, there appears to be an increasing number of 'cultures' and 'imagined communities' emerging with the growth of global diasporas, that are leading to globally based localisation as well as increasing numbers of localities that are geographically based but not necessarily culturally determined. With increasing specialisation, as a feature of late modernity and globalisation, leading to fragmentation, the question must be – how is the conduct of childbirth changing around the world in response to globalisation and what consequences does this hold for women in childbirth?

In this book I explore the context of childbirth, and attempt to uncover how the balances of power between competing discourses construct, negotiate and control, and in some instances impose, what is accepted as the cultural commonsense of birthing practice in specific environments.

Our inability to come to terms with childbirth systems failure stems from the fact that television reduces political discourse to sound bites and that academia and medicine organise scientific and intellectual inquiry into narrowly specialised disciplines. As a result we become accustomed to dealing with complex issues, such as childbirth, in fragmented components. Yet in the complex world in which we live nearly every aspect of our lives is connected in some way with every other aspect. Consequently, if we limit ourselves to fragmented approaches to dealing with universal problems or natural physiological events such as birth, it is not surprising that our solutions prove inadequate. If as human beings we are to survive the predicaments we have created for ourselves, a capacity for whole-systems thought and action must be developed. Whole-systems thought must include the environment, culture, politics, issues of power and control, institutions and so on.

Whole-systems thinking calls for a scepticism of simplistic solutions, a willingness to seek out connections between problems and events that conventional discourse ignores, and the courage to delve into subject matter that may lie outside our direct experience and expertise (Korten, 1995: 11).

In taking a whole-systems perspective, this book explores a broad terrain with many elements. To help the reader keep in mind how the individual arguments that are developed and documented throughout the book link together into a larger whole, the overall argument is summarised here. It must be borne in mind, however, that we are all participants in an act of creation, and none of us can claim a monopoly on truth in our individual and collective search for understanding of these complex issues.

The point of departure for *Childbirth in the Global Village* is the evidence that we are experiencing accelerating social and environmental disintegration in nearly every country of the world, as manifested by increases in poverty, unemployment, inequality, violent crime, failing families, and environmental degradation. These problems stem in part from a massive increase in economic output over the past fifty years that has forced demands on the ecosystem beyond that which the planet is capable of sustaining. For Korten, the continued drive for economic growth as the organising principle of public policy is accelerating the breakdown of the ecosystem's regenerative capacities. Moreover, the social fabric that sustains human community is under threat. At the same time, it is intensifying the competition for resources between rich and poor, a competition that the poor invariably lose (ibid.).

According to Wilkinson (2000) it is clear now that our health is overwhelmingly affected not so much by medical care as by the social and economic circumstances in which people live. Many influences on our health are subtler than diet and exercise for example. It is now apparent that some of the most important links between our health and living conditions are psychosocial, that is, many of the biological processes leading to illness or complications of pregnancy and childbirth are triggered by our subjective experiences of life. Socio-economic inequality exerts profound effects on the quality of the social environment and the psychosocial welfare of the population. The relationship between income inequality and characteristics of the social environment such as friendships, trust, involvement in community life, hostility and violent crime, are strong. As a society becomes more unequal and hierarchical, the quality of social relations and friendship deteriorates (with more violence and less trust). Wilkinson noted that hierarchy and social relations are closely related to each other in an important way: 'it is not just that social relations worsen when societies are more hierarchical – intriguingly, both factors are powerfully related to health.' (2000: 16). Weak social affiliations and low social class are among the most important risk factors affecting health globally.

A large proportion of the population in most countries around the world is exposed to the difficulties of subordinate social status. When combined with poor social networks and vast differences in health equality, social status – an increasing feature of American and British society according to Putnam (2000) – becomes an important determinant of health. Indeed, for Wilkinson (2000: 17) 'there could hardly be a more harmful mix for population health than widening differences in social status and a simultaneous atrophying of friendship networks.'

Against this backcloth, women are struggling to give birth while large global organisations are spreading simplistic solutions to health problems based on economic equations and Western medical ideologies. Western concepts regarding childbirth are being exchanged across the world with the result that these solutions are being exported, perhaps without any real analysis of the issues. Medical ideology, using measurement and concepts of risk and probability, is altering the ways in which childbirth is conducted in traditional societies, not always to their benefit. The problems within the medical systems in the West are being carried over into the developing world. At the same time in the more advanced societies, concepts of continuity and community are emerging as idealised approaches to birth derived from those very communities who are now being encouraged to abandon them.

Those who bear the costs of the system's dysfunction have been stripped of decision-making power and are held in a state of confusion regarding the cause of their distress by corporate-dominated media that incessantly bombards them with interpretations of the resulting crisis based on the perceptions of the power holders. An active propaganda machine controlled by the world's largest organisations including the World Bank, World Health Organization and other non-governmental organisations constantly propagates myths to justify the spread of the dominant Western medical ideology. This effectively masks the extent to which the global transformation of human institutions at local and national levels is a consequence of the sophisticated, well-funded, and intentional interventions of a small elite. Their money enables them to live in a world of illusion apart from the rest of humanity.

This in turn affects the way that the local culture and location of birthing fits with global perspectives and midwives' personal beliefs about birth, women and midwifery practice. This is not a book about results, but about processes. The women who appear in these pages continue to act and react, shaping and being shaped by the transformation that characterises their world. In so doing, they manage to face inherent conflicts and contradictions and to devise compromises and accommodations that permit them to develop new strategies. I have caught them at one moment in time but they continue to balance their lives in a world that continues to change.

In the following chapters the backcloth of women's lives in the global village and the impact of modernity, development strategies and risk are examined before exploring the experience and context of childbirth in Africa, Malaysia, America and England.

Chapter 4 presents vignettes of the experience of women in childbirth and the women who attend them in Ghana and Malawi. Both countries are in a phase of development and can be found along the continuum of pre-modern to modern, but largely maintain their traditional, pre-modern, albeit colonial-influenced, cultures.

In chapter 5 the journey moves to Malaysia where the context of childbirth and the social situation of women is rapidly changing. Malaysia typifies a country in a transitional phase of development and women are forced to realign their concepts and beliefs about themselves, their role and childbirth as the country passes into modernity.

In chapter 6 we journey from a transitional culture to one that can be described as the most modern country in the world – the United States of America – where women in childbirth are also experiencing change as the medical profession increasingly introduces more complex technology into the birthing context. Birth technology is also a feature in British childbirth and in chapter 7 the experience of women in England is explored as they try to balance 'risk' with notions of 'safety'.

The key elements of the case studies are drawn together and reflected upon in chapter 8 where the cultural implications of science and mathematics on childbirth and notions of risk and making motherhood safe are discussed.

In chapter 9 the cultural implications of globalisation for education and training of practitioners in childbirth are explored before discussing the implications of the curricula approaches to practitioner development. The final chapter draws the threads of the book to a conclusion.

Chapter 2

The global village

This chapter explores a number of significant global issues pertinent to the study of women in childbirth. The issues addressed here have been categorised into specific 'globalscapes' concerned with the media and communication, culture, globality and locality, technology, the environment, the exchange of symbols that work to globalise, and the cultural alignments people make within the global village. Contained within these categories are a number of key issues that impact upon individuals and their lifestyles.

Whilst each category identifies a specific area for elaboration, it is important to emphasise that they are all interdependent and interactive. Thus it is difficult to entirely separate actions undertaken in one area from their impact on another. As a result, none of the categories has a hierarchical position over any other and therefore they are not presented here in an order that represents their importance.

Globalisation has fuelled a boom in political, economic, and environmental debate and academic publication over the past two decades. The processes that these debates represent have been in evidence for quite some time, longer than is implied by the manner in which the concept of globalisation is sometimes used. Some of the dimensions of what is currently described as globalisation have been a feature of human activities for centuries. They can be discerned, for example, in the excitement which attended the introduction of technologies in the nineteenth and early twentieth centuries, including the telegraph, telephone, radio, photography and film. The globalisation process today is marked by the accelerated pace at which informational and cultural exchanges take place and by the scale and complexity of these exchanges (on the latter, see Appadurai, 1990: 6). They include the increasing volume and international flavour of the goods that are available to the public, international tourism and migration, internationalisation of ownership of property and businesses, shared possession and use of media products and icons across national boundaries. The global availability of a wide range of moving images in films and television programmes, press and magazine articles, photography and music is difficult to ignore.

Facilitated by the new technologies, it is the sheer speed, extent and volume of these exchanges and their effect on everyday life that have engaged popular imagination. Cheater (1993: 3–4) lists an impressive array of such technologies, from electronic mail to the satellite dish, which although not accessible to all, have been directly or indirectly responsible for exposing many different sorts of people to new influences. Such technologies are able to uncouple culture from its territorial base so that, detached and unanchored, it travels through the airwaves to all those with the means to receive it. The accelerating effects of electronic communication and rapid transportation that can whisk people from one location to another create a structural effect that McLuhan (1964: 185) called 'implosion'. By this he meant the bringing together in one place of all aspects of experience, a place where one can simultaneously sense and touch events and objects that are great distances apart. The centre-margin structure of industrial civilisation disappears in the face of global synchronised and instantaneous experience. In what has become an evocative and iconic formulation, McLuhan asserted 'This is the New World of the global village' (ibid.: 93). But global space is not in any way similar to a tribal village.

The debates about globalisation cross many disciplines. For example, Giddens (1990) firmly situated globalisation as a consequence of modernity, whose dynamics radically transform social relations across time and space. More specifically, he argued that globalisation occurs in four key domains: the extension of the nation-state system; the global reach of the capitalist economy coupled with the international division of labour; and a global system of military alliances. Robertson (1992) anchors the development of globalisation in an earlier history and outlines a five-phase model in which many more institutions, actors and ideological and cultural elements play a role. Hannerz (1990) argued that the assumption common to much globalisation discourse, as also to preceding theories of cultural and media imperialism before it, that globalisation and its cultures moves from the 'centre' (that is, the West) towards the periphery in largely one way flows was erroneous. He argued that centre-periphery relations are much more complex; cultural flows can and do move in multiple directions. This tension is reflected in the many contributions on globalisation. The central question is whether there can be a global society. Such a development would be more than just the sum of the parts (global economic relations, global political institutions, and a shared globalised culture); it would be based around new forms of identification.

Globalization and its derivations (globality, globalism, etc.) are metaphors that capture a disparate range of phenomena and experiences. The global metaphor has an important significance for broadly indicating the actual range of human activities across the world while, at the same time, disregarding any divisions that human beings might establish between themselves.

The increasing interdependence of national economies – as well as increasing social and cultural global linkages – means that economic fluctuations and their social impacts now reverberate on a global level. Growing poverty and insecurity are linked to social conflict, extremism, violence, crime, child labour and other social problems. Because the source of these problems involves a global dimension, their solutions cannot be found only on the local level: local and national action must be complemented by action taken at the global level.

Symbolic exchanges

Waters (1995) argued that globalisation resulted primarily from the exchange of symbols. For him, globalisation proceeds much more rapidly in contexts in which relationships are mediated through symbols and rituals. Economic globalisation is therefore most advanced in the financial markets that are mediated by monetary tokens and to the extent that production is dematerialised. Political globalisation has advanced to the extent that there is an appreciation of common global values and problems rather than commitments to material interests. However, material and power exchanges are rapidly becoming displaced by symbolic exchanges, that is, by relationships based on values, preferences and tastes rather than by material inequality and constraint. In the context of this argument, globalisation might be seen as an aspect of the progressive 'culturalisation' of social life (Waters, 1995: 124).

A globalised culture is chaotic rather than orderly – it is integrated and connected so that the meanings of its components are 'relativised' to one another but it is not unified or centralised. The absolute globalisation of culture would involve the creation of a common but hyper-differentiated field of value, taste, and style opportunities, accessible by each individual without constraint for purposes either of self-expression or consumption.

The concept of globalisation is an obvious object, claimed Waters (ibid.: 3), for ideological suspicion because, like modernisation, a predecessor and related concept, it appears to justify the spread of Western culture and of capitalist society by suggesting that there are forces beyond human control that are transforming the world. This book makes no attempt to hide the fact that the current phase of globalisation as it impacts on women in childbirth, is precisely associated with these developments. Globalization is the direct consequence of the expansion of European and American culture across the planet via settlement, colonisation, and cultural imitation.

For Waters (1995), the contemporary accelerated pace of globalisation is directly attributable to the explosion in signs and symbols. Human society is globalising to the extent that human relationships and institutions can be converted from experience to information, to the extent it is arranged in space around consumption of symbols rather than the production of material goods, to the extent that value-commitments are badges of identity, to the extent that politics is the pursuit of lifestyle, and to the extent that organisational constraints and political surveillance are displaced in favour of reflexive self-examination. These and other cultural forces have become so overwhelming that they have breached the banks not only of national value-systems but also of industrial organisations and political-territorial arrangements. Globalisation does not imply, however, that every part of the world has become westernised and capitalist, rather, those social arrangements in every sector must establish their position in relation to the capitalist West.

Friedman (1999: 7) agreed with this analysis and argued further that globalisation is the international system that replaced the Cold War system. For him, the Cold War system was defined by a single word – division – and it was symbolised by a single object – a wall, the Berlin Wall. It was a divided world in which one could not go very far or very fast in this world without running into a wall.

The globalised world is also defined by a single word – integration. All the threats and opportunities in this globalised world flow from integration and it is symbolised not by a wall but by a virtual object – the World Wide Web, which provides the opportunity to unite everyone. Friedman considered that we no longer have a first, second or third world, rather there is just a fast world and a slow world. The globalisation system, unlike the Cold War system, is not static, but a dynamic ongoing process that involves the inexorable integration of markets, nation-states, and technologies to a degree never seen before. This is happening in a way that is enabling individuals, corporations and nation-states to reach around the world farther, faster, deeper, and cheaper than ever before. Friedman equates globalisation to running in the hundred-metre dash run over and over and over again, and no matter how many times you win, you have to race again the next day. If you lose by one tenth of a second, it is as if you lose by two hours. The widening gap can, and does, result in a powerful backlash from those brutalised or left behind by this new system. For example, in many countries where the International Monetary Fund (IMF) and World Bank have imposed structural adjustment programs (SAPs), the people who have seen deterioration in their standards of living, reduced access to public services, devastated environments, and plummeting employment prospects have not been passive. The pages of newspapers, magazines, and academic journals that survive in depressed economies, have been filled with damning analyses of structural adjustment. More important, people have been organising themselves to combat the pillaging of their lands and livelihoods. This organising has resulted in mass movements and protests on every continent, but they are not often reported on in the mainstream press. The following example illustrates the level of concern raised by countries subject to restructuring.

Zambia: April 2000

Scores of anti-IMF protesters dispersed by armed riot police in Zambia's capital Lusaka after they attempted to picket outside a hotel where IMF and Zambian officials were meeting. 'IMF policies are killing us, especially women and children,' said a representative of one of the many women's groups that organized the protest.

(*Sonoma County Peace Press*, 2000)

Waters (1995: 7), argued that globalisation can be traced through three arenas of social life that have come to be recognised as fundamental in many theoretical analyses (for example, see Abercrombie, 1980/90, Aharoni, 1993, Appadurai, 1990, Bader, 1979, Boyne, 1990, Cockerham, 1995, Dezalay, 1990, Gessner and Schade, 1990, Featherstone, 1990, Friedman, 1999, Giddens, 1989, 1990, Hannerz, 1990, King, 1990, Robertson, 1992, Wallerstein, 1989, Worsley, 1990). These are:

1 *The economy* Social arrangements for the production, exchange, distribution and consumption of goods and tangible services.

For Freidman (1999) the driving idea behind globalisation is the spread of free-market capitalism to every country in the world under the belief that the more market forces rule and the more the economy is open to free trade and competition, the more efficient and flourishing the economy will be. Along with its own set of economic rules that revolve around opening, deregulating and privatising the economy, globalisation also has its own defining technologies: computerisation, miniaturisation, digitisation, satellite communications, fibre optics and the Internet. These technologies help to create the defining perspective of globalisation. Moreover, these technologies act as symbols of the modern world.

Since capitalism has been (and continues to be) a revolutionary mode of production in which the material practices and processes of social reproduction are always changing, it follows that the objective qualities as well as the meanings of space and time also change. On the other hand, if advances in knowledge (scientific, technical, administrative, bureaucratic, and rational) are vital to the progress of capitalist production and consumption, then changes in our conceptual apparatus (including representations of time and space) can have material consequences for the ordering of daily life, including childbirth.

This does not mean that practices are determined by formulae for they have the awkward habit of escaping their moorings in any fixed scheme of representation. New meanings can be found for older materialisation of space and time. We appropriate ancient spaces in very modern ways, treat time and history as something to create rather than accept. The same concept of community, as a social entity created in space through time, can disguise radical differences in meaning because the processes of community production themselves diverge remarkably according to group capacities and interests. Yet treatment of communities as if they are comparable by, for example, a planning agency, has material implications to which the social practices of people who live in them have to respond. Beneath the veneer of common sense and seemingly 'natural' ideas about time and space, there lie hidden terrains of ambiguity, contradiction and struggle. Conflicts arise not merely out of admittedly diverse subjective appreciation, but because different objective material qualities of time and space are deemed relevant to social life in different situations.

Harvey (1992: 205) argued that important battles likewise occur in the realms of scientific, social, and aesthetic theory, as well as in practice. How we represent time and space in theory matters because it affects how others, and we interpret and then act with respect to the world.

2 The polity Social arrangements for the concentration and application of power, especially insofar as it involves the organised exchange of coercion and surveillance (military, police, etc.) as well as such institutionalised transactions of these practices as authority and diplomacy, that can establish control over populations and territories.

Most importantly, globalisation has its own defining complex structure of power. The Cold War system was built exclusively around nation-states, and it was balanced at the centre by two superpowers: the United States and the Soviet Union. For Friedman (1999: 11) the globalised system, by contrast, is built around three overlapping and interacting balances – the nation-state (i.e. the superpower), the multinational companies, or the supermarkets, and, in Friedman's terms, the relatively unrecognised, the super-empowered individual.

The first is the traditional balance between nation-states. In the globalised system, the United States of America is now the dominant superpower and all other nations are subordinate to it to one degree or another. The balance of power between the United States and the other states is still important for the stability of this system. The second balance in the globalisation system is between nation-states and global markets. These global markets comprise investors moving money around the world by a click of a 'mouse'. Friedman refers to them as 'the Electronic Herd'. This herd gathers in key global financial centres, such as Wall Street, Hong Kong, London and Frankfurt, which he calls 'the Supermarkets.' The attitudes and actions of the electronic herd and the supermarkets can have a significant impact on nation-states today, even to the point of triggering the downfall of governments.

The United States is the dominant player in maintaining the globalisation 'gameboard' (Friedman, ibid.: 12). But it is not alone in influencing the moves on that gameboard. Sometimes pieces are moved around by the obvious hand of the superpower, and sometimes the invisible hands of the supermarkets move them around.

The third balance in the globalisation system is the balance between individuals and nation-states. Since globalisation has eliminated many of the boundaries that restricted the movement and reach of people, and because it has simultaneously networked the world, it gives more power to individuals to influence both markets and nation-states than at any other time in history. Consequently, there are now not only a superpower and supermarkets, but also super-empowered individuals able to act directly on the world stage without the traditional mediation of governments, corporations or any other public or private institutions. For example, Jodie Williams who won the Nobel Peace Prize in 1997 for her contribution to the International Ban on Landmines achieved that ban not only without much government help, but also in the face of opposition from the Big Five major powers. Her secret weapon for organising 1,000 different human rights and arms control groups on six continents was simply 'e-mail' (Friedman, ibid.: 13).

Nation-states, and the American superpower in particular, are still hugely important today, but so too now are supermarkets and super-empowered individuals. To understand the globalisation system, it is vital to 'see it as a complex interaction between all three of these actors: states bumping up against states, states bumping up against supermarkets, and supermarkets and states bumping up against super-empowered individuals' (Friedman, ibid.: 13).

3 Culture Social arrangements for the production, exchange and expression of symbols that represent facts, affects, meanings, beliefs, preferences, tastes and values.

> In my travels around the globe it seemed to me that Western culture has penetrated even the most remote areas. This appears to be mainly through a process of media communication. When visiting a remote village in Ghana I saw a young child wearing a t-shirt proclaiming Coca-Cola to be the 'best'. On questioning the level of understanding of the meaning of the advertisement, the child revealed that Coca-Cola was delivered to the local store. This local store was a wooden one room shack on the side of the road in the village.

The emergence of large international media companies which own media interests in numerous countries increasingly functions to undermine any sense of a national media tied to a particular nation-state. Their interests are global and they have done much to generate international markets rather than national markets for their products, particularly promoting new technologies such as satellite, which have no national boundaries. They have benefited from the general deregulation and the marketisation of modern culture in the last two decades. There has been what Thompson (1990, chapter 4) terms the 'mediatization' of culture (see also Brunn and Leinback, 1991). Against such obvious power of these companies, it is a relatively simple matter to hypothesise the weakness of individual consumers. It seems uncontroversial to suggest that the effect will be to produce mass consumers of the products of such companies on a world scale.

Patterns of social interaction and information flows are increasingly occurring across national boundaries to form new bases of social, political and cultural identity. Communication networks, previously responsible for vertical integration of a society, are stimulating emerging patterns of social interaction and political organisation, changing ideological assumptions and cultural forms as well as information flows, transitionally in a process of horizontal integration and articulation.

Once a country makes the leap into the system of globalisation, its elites begin to internalise this perspective of integration, and will always try to locate themselves in a global context. Unlike the Cold War system, globalisation has its own dominant culture, which is why it tends to be homogenising. In previous eras this sort of cultural homogenisation happened on a regional scale. Friedman (1999: 8) gives the examples of the Turkification of Central Asia, North Africa, Europe and the Middle East by the Ottomans or the Russification of Eastern and Central Europe and parts of Eurasia under the Soviets. Culturally speaking, in his view, globalisation is largely, though not entirely, the spread of Americanism.

Globalization is also characterised by its own demographic pattern exemplified by the rapid acceleration of the movement of people from rural areas and agricultural lifestyles to urban areas and urban lifestyles that are more intimately associated with global consumerist trends in fashion, music, food, and entertainment.

Waters (1995) takes the three arenas of the economy, polity and culture to be structurally independent. The argument, however, does make the assumption that the relative effectiveness of the arenas can vary across history and geography. A set of arrangements, perceived to be more effective in one arena can penetrate and modify arrangements in the others just as a more effective set of arrangements in one country can penetrate and modify arrangements in another. Changes in the practice and rituals of childbirth are one example of this.

These themes can now be linked to an argument about globalisation. Waters argued that the types of exchange that predominate establish the link between social organisation and territoriality in social relationships at any particular moment. Different types of exchanges in his view apply to each of the arenas indicated above. Respectively these are:

- material exchanges including trade, tenancy, wage-labour, fee-for-service and capital accumulation;
- political exchanges of support, security, coercion, authority, force, surveillance, legitimacy and obedience;
- symbolic exchanges by means of oral communication, publication, performance, teaching, oratory, ritual, display, entertainment, propaganda,

advertisement, public demonstration, data accumulation and transfer (research), exhibition and spectacle.

For Waters (ibid.: 9) each of these exchanges exhibit a particular relationship to space.

- Material exchanges tend to tie social relationships to localities: the production of exchangeable items involves local concentrations of labour, capital and raw materials; commodities are costly to transport which mitigates against long-distance trade unless there are significant cost advantages; wage-labour involves face-to-face supervision; service delivery is also most often face-to-face. Material exchanges are therefore rooted in localised markets, factories and shops. Specialist intermediaries (merchants, sailors, financiers, etc.) who stand outside the central relationship of the economy are required to carry out long-distance trade.
- Political exchanges tend to tie relationships to extended territories. They are specifically directed towards controlling the population that occupies a territory and harnessing its resources in the direction of territorial integrity or expansion. Political exchanges therefore culminate in the establishment of territorial boundaries that are coterminous with nation-state societies. The exchanges between these units, known as international relations (i.e. war and diplomacy), tend to confirm their territorial sovereignty.
- Symbolic exchanges liberate relationships from spatial referents. Symbols can be produced anywhere and at any time and there are relatively few resource constraints on their production and reproduction. Moreover they are easily transportable. Importantly, because they frequently seek to appeal to human fundamentals they can also claim universal significance.

It follows that the globalisation of human society is contingent on the extent to which cultural arrangements are effective relative to economic and political arrangements. Waters expects the economy and the polity to be globalised to the extent that they are culturalised, that is, to the extent that the exchanges that take place within them are accomplished symbolically. We would also expect that the degree of globalisation is greater in the cultural arena than either of the other two.

Reflexive modernity

Symbolic tokens, according to Giddens, are for the most part concerned with money tokens. Such tokens have enabled the extension of reach across national and local boundaries. While expert systems represent the repositories of technical knowledge that can be deployed across a wide range of actual contexts. Expert systems provide guarantees about what to expect across all of these contexts and ultimately lead to standardisation and routinisation of activity. Both imply an attitude of trust. That is, people have to have confidence in the value of money and technology and the accuracy of expertise that is provided by absent others. Modernity, therefore, implies a high level of trust alongside high risk.

The fact that modern people trust their societies and their lives to be guided by impersonal flows of money and expertise does not necessarily mean that they leave all decision making to others. Modern people engage in monitoring activities because they are aware of risk. People do constantly observe, inquire about and consider the value of money and the validity of expertise. Modern society is therefore, for Giddens (1990), reflexive in character. Social activity is constantly informed by flows of information and analysis that subject it to continuous revision and thereby constitute and reproduce it. 'Knowing what to do' in modern society, even in such traditional contexts as kinship and childbirth, almost always involves acquiring knowledge about how it is done from books, television programmes or experts in the specialist field, rather than relying on experience of self and others or the authoritarian knowledge of elders.

The particular difficulties faced by modern people are that this knowledge is constantly and rapidly changing so that living in a modern society appears to be uncontrolled or chaotic. The proliferation of knowledge and symbols promotes two kinds of reflexivity.

- It promotes a pattern of what Lash and Urry (1994) refer to as 'reflexive accumulation', the individualised self-monitoring of production and of expertise and an accompanying increasing and widespread tendency to question authority and expertise.
- It promotes an aesthetic or expressive reflexivity in which individuals constantly reference self-presentation in relation to a normalised set of possible meanings given in the increasing flow of symbols. People monitor their own images and deliberately alter them. These images may fall into four different cultural types.

Cultural types

According to Douglas (1997: 18) and Thompson (1992: 182–198) there are four distinctive ways of organising modern society. These four cultures, as Douglas terms them, are each in conflict with the others. People tend to embody one of the cultures and play out a lifestyle that exemplifies that cultural type as exemplified in the following descriptions expounded by Thompson (ibid.).

Individualistic or entrepreneurial lifestyle

Those subscribing to this cultural type tend to be characterised as 'driving in the fast lane'. They tend to be entrepreneurial, competitive with wide flung, open ego-focused networks of people. They enjoy high tech instruments and generally lead a risky lifestyle, insisting on the freedom to change commitments. Persons who subscribe to this cultural lifestyle are on the whole knowledgeable, enthusiastic and fashion conscious (even to the most fashionable way of giving birth). The individualist's philosophy of life and cultural bias embraces politics, aesthetics, religion, morals, friendships, food and hygiene. They have a cosmopolitan, neophiliac and wide-ranging consumption style. For them, nature is benign and they view resources as being abundant. The individualist perception of time is that short term dominates long term and they have a preference for laissez-faire governance. Their commitment to the organisation only lasts as long as it is profitable to the individual. The individualist cultural alignment is based on a way of life that is free to bid and bargain and needs nature and women to be robust to refute arguments of those who are against any action s/he has in mind. If things go wrong either the unproductive individual or the external distortions of the market get the blame.

Hierarchical lifestyle

Persons subscribing to this cultural type are characterised as being formal; adhering to established traditions and established institutions. They insist on maintaining a defined network of family and friends (driving in the slow lane). They view their knowledge as almost complete and organised. For them nature is robust, but only within limits. This lifestyle justifies the hierarchist's control of nature and the environment through the institution of regulations and procedures on the individualist's projects. Their solution to 'pollution' (and here pollution can also be understood as deviation from the expected norm of society) is to change nature to conform to society (this is most clearly manifested in the control of childbirth). The hierarchist consumption style is essentially traditional with strong links to the past and others within the group. The hierarchist favours 'high tech' virtuosity on a large scale and is biased toward ritualism and sacrifice in order to maintain control. They view resources as scarce and prefer bureaucratisation through increasing transaction costs. For them the greatest risk lies in the loss of control (i.e. public trust). Their commitment to institutions takes the form of correct procedures and discriminated statuses that are supported for their own sake. Their watchword is 'loyalty'. Women in childbirth within this lifestyle need structure. If things go wrong, the 'victim' gets the blame.

Enclavist or egalitarian lifestyle

The enclavist is essentially egalitarian and is against formality, pomp and artifice. Enclavists reject authoritarian institutions, preferring simplicity, frankness, intimate friendships and spiritual values. Nature and women are ephemeral, fragile and pollution (either physical or spiritual) can be lethal. Their knowledge is viewed as imperfect but holistic. This lifestyle is in fundamental disagreement with the policies of the development entre-preneurs (individualist) and with the organising hierarchists, and with the fatalism of the isolate. They see resources as depleting and lean towards a frugal and environmentally benign approach to technology and industry. They consider that society needs to conform to nature, consequently, their cultural bias favours fundamentalism (not necessarily in a religious sense) and millenarianism. Their preferred economic theory verges on Buddhist and thermo-dynamic approaches to economics. For them the long-term concerns dominate short-term activities and gains. The egalitarian views the risks associated with global development strategies as catastrophic, irreversible and inequitable. Their commitment to institutions takes the form of collect-ive moral fervour and affirmation of shared opposition to the outside world. Their watchword is 'voice'. Women in childbirth in this lifestyle need to be activists. If things go wrongs, the system gets the blame.

Isolate or fatalist lifestyle

This refers to a lifestyle that is characterised as eclectic, withdrawn but unpredictable along with a refusal to be recruited to any cause. Friends do not impose upon the isolate, and s/he is not hassled by competition or burdened by obligatory gifts, nor irritated by tight arrangements or timetables. In this cultural type, nature and women are seen as unpredictable and capricious. The isolate takes a fatalistic approach to life and views the acquisition of resources as a lottery. The scope of knowledge is irrelevant and learning is a matter of luck. Their priority is to cope with the chaos of daily life, the survival of the individual is the paramount concern, and thus they devise short-term responses to cope with erratic mismatches of needs and resources. Their con-sumption style is isolated and traditionalist but they have weak connections to past or others. The isolationist often has low productivity but is highly innova-tive. If things go wrong, 'it's the poor that gets the blame'. Women in child-birth in this lifestyle are marginalised through structural imbalance. They need to maintain their dignity through acceptance of their situation.

To understand the way in which our social experience affects how we think we need to recognise two distinct ways in which society may exert pressure on an individual, two distinct ways in which society may restrict his/her options. Douglas (1992: 9) uses the term 'grid' to refer to restrictions that arise from the system of social classification, for example, the distinction between lord and commoner or between man and woman. Grid in this sense is the set of rules, which govern individuals in their personal interactions. Strong or 'high' grid means strongly defined roles, which provide a script for individual interaction. Towards the weak end of this axis, the public signals of rank and status fade and ambiguity enters the relationships. Individuals no longer have the guidance of a script, but are valued as individuals and relate to each other as such. The constraints become correspondingly weaker, until they take only the generalised form of respect for each person as a unique individual.

Douglas uses the term 'group' to refer to the extent to which an individual's interactions are confined within a specific group of people who form a sub-group within the larger community. Where the group is strong, there is a clear boundary between members and non-members, and though it may be possible for an individual to leave the group that will have high costs in that membership of the group confers benefits. Consider the case of Wendy Savage (1986), for example, who risked alienating herself from the dominant obstetric group by advocating different approaches to childbirth. As a result, members of the group are able to exert considerable pressure on the individual to conform to its requirements. By contrast, where the group is weak, the individual is free to form relationships or negotiate exchanges with anyone, and the resulting network of interactions constitutes a myriad of overlapping groups, with sub-groups of individuals who interact only with themselves.

Cultural theory and myths of childbirth

Douglas' (1966) and Turner's (1969) concept of ritual as stereotyped actions that remain faithful to an established cultural pattern can explain the cultural dynamics of the ritualised processes of childbirth, in part. The invariability of these processes grants them efficacy in many different domains, ranging from promoting social solidarity, order, purity, health or fertility to effecting changes of status, to causing harm to someone. Moreover, it is precisely through this changeless nature that rites play an important role in complementing the information provided by mythology. The link to mythology is so close that it can be said that rites are the enactment of myths.

Rites are commonly divided into two kinds: public and private. Public rites are concerned with social groups bigger than those of the individual, family or domestic unit. The setting for these rituals is often a village, compound, school or hospital, for example. Private rites are more to do with the individual or family. Rituals have several phases (see van Gennep, 1966; Turner, 1969), which alternate between liminal and structured periods. Consequently, in addition to examining the symbols that surround rites one also needs to have regard to their sequence. Moreover, since the actions take place in particular areas and among people who have some kind of relationship, spatial referents and social relationships also provide important information. Through them one can obtain information about conceptions of space and time and about patterns of social interaction.

Conclusion

Having considered the various explanations and definitions offered by a multiplicity of authors, globalisation, for me, is a metaphor that encapsulates a variety of different elements, processes and actions. It is an unfolding story over time that illustrates the seeming compression of the world through the transcendence of national boundaries and the intensification of consciousness of the world as a whole. It conveys a widespread sense of transformation of the world by expanding the frontiers of relevance beyond the narrow time and spatial boundaries of modernity, thus reintroducing grand narrative that brings history into the present.

The creation of the global village through globalisation is the making or the experience of being made, global at the individual level by the active dissemination of practices, values, technology and other human products throughout the globe. The global village is manifest when global practices exercise an increasing influence over people's lives, when the globe serves as a focus for, or as a premise on which to shape human activities. In practice, however, there is no inherent logic to globalisation that suggests a particular outcome will prevail. Globalisation is, therefore, ultimately indeterminate and ambiguous.

Taken together, the theories of globalisation represent a new sociology of globalisation that has emerged over the past two decades. In summary, it proposes that:

- Globalisation is at least contemporary with modernisation and therefore has been proceeding for the past three centuries. It involves processes of economic systemisation, international relations and an emerging global culture. The process has accelerated through time and is currently in a highly rapid phase of its development.
- Globalisation increases the inclusiveness and the unification of human society by involving the systematic interrelationship of all individual social ties. No relationship can remain isolated or bounded in a fully globalised context. Each is linked to the others and is systematically affected by them especially in a territorial sense where geographical boundaries are unsustainable in the face of globalisation.
- Globalisation involves a phenomenology of contraction – time-space compression – in which the world appears to be shrinking.
- The phenomenology of globalisation is reflexive (Giddens, 1991). People orientate themselves to the world as a whole – multinational companies explore global markets, countercultures move from an 'alternative

community' to a 'social movement' and governments attempt to maintain a level of human rights and will often intervene to maintain world order (take the more recent conflicts in Kosovo (UNHCR, 1999; United Nations, 2000).

- Globalisation involves a collapse of the differentiation between public and private spaces, work and home and system and lifeworld. The separation was largely accomplished by boundaries in time and space but because globalisation annihilates time and space the distinctions can no longer apply. Each person in any relationship is simultaneously an individual and a member of human society.
- Globalisation involves a Janus-faced mix of risk and trust (Giddens, 1991). Giddens argued that in previous eras people trusted the immediate, the knowable, the present and the material. To go beyond these is to run the risk of injury or exploitation. Under globalisation individuals extend trust to unknown persons, to impersonal forces and norms (the 'market', or 'human rights') and to patterns of symbolic exchange that appear to be beyond the control of any concrete individual or group of individuals. In so doing they place themselves in the hands of their fellow human beings. Consequently, the commitment of all the participants is necessary for the wellbeing of each individual member.
- Each individual 'buys' into a lifestyle that best exemplifies their personal values and beliefs about the social, cultural, environmental, political and financial world.

For Albrow (1996: 95–96) we have moved from the Modern Age to the Global Age. He believes that we have not realised the profundity of this break as yet. For that to happen, he claims, we need to look crucially at the narrative habits behind which modernity has sought to conceal the demise of the Modern Age. But are we, as yet, ready to deny the real experiences of modernity that we encounter daily? In order to be ready to discard the idea of the passing of the Modern Age we need to first explore what is meant by the terms 'modern', 'modernity', 'modernisation' and all their derivatives, all of which will be considered in the next chapter.

Chapter 3

The nature of modernity

Society, development and risk

Engagement in modernisation and industrialisation effects permanent changes on a country and its people. For traditional societies, life was, and is, determined by natural forces in combination with forces of spiritual necessities. People functioned, and continue to function, in accordance with the natural laws of seasons, sunrise and sunset, low tide and high tide. Their lives mostly revolved around locally determined material exchanges of goods and services. Religion and traditional belief systems prescribed the course of everyday life.

Industrialisation carries with it general societal ramifications. It induces the pattern of differentiation in a number of areas of social life as these increasingly become functionally articulated with the industrial core, for example, the movement of childbirth and health care from home to hospital. Families specialise in consumption, schools teach differentiated skills to the labour force, specialised units of government provide economic infrastructure, the mass media sell appropriate symbolic representations of the world, churches promulgate supporting values, and so on.

These structural changes induce value shifts in the direction of individualisation, universalism, secularity and rationalisation. This general complex of transformations is 'modernisation.' As industrialisation spreads across the globe, it carries modernisation with it, transforming societies in a unitary direction. Imitating societies may even adopt modern institutions before effectively industrialising.

Levy (1966) defined modernisation in the following way: 'A society will be considered more or less modernised to the extent that its members use inanimate sources of power and/or use tools to multiply the effects of their efforts' (1966: 11). Such is the case in childbirth in the United States of America and the United Kingdom. Increasingly this is evolving as the situation in major urban centres in Malaysia, Ghana and Malawi. Levy also lists the major societal-structural characteristics of a relatively modern society (1966: 38–79). Many of these bear a close resemblance to Parsons' (1964) evolutionary universals:

- The units of society, its collectivities and roles are highly specialised with respect to the type of activity, which they perform; this means that individuals can specialise in the skills, which they use in role performance.
- The units of society have a relatively low level of self-sufficiency – they must rely on other units to provide resources which they do not themselves produce.
- Value-orientations are highly universalistic – they tend to stress what a person can do that is relevant to the situation rather than what they are.
- An increasing centralisation of decision-making is set up by the need to coordinate and control diverse, specialised activities.
- A large proportion of human relationships are characterised by rationality, universalism, functional specificity and emotional avoidance.
- A large proportion of the exchanges between specialised units takes place by means of generalised media (e.g. money) and within market contexts.
- The multilineal, conjugal family is established, which covers a maximum of two generations, disemphasises unilineal descent, and focuses on the spouse relationship as the foundational bond.

Modernisation in these terms is no longer the impersonal functional imperative of adaptive upgrading (Parsons, 1964) but rather a materialistic motivation at the level of the individual agent. Once a traditional society is in contact with a modernised society, at least some of its members will want to change it in order to improve their material situation, more or less out of envy of the 'inordinate material productivity' of modern societies (Levy, 1966: 125–6).

Social consequences of adjustment and restructuring

It is generally assumed that the development of a society depends on the improvement of the socio-economic conditions, i.e. on economic growth and the improvement of existing, and the invention of new, technologies to rationalise production processes and services. Research and development play a key role in driving the economic sectors of industrialised societies. The production of knowledge and skills to develop, implement and control technologies lies at the heart of these societies. While traditional societies are based on agriculture, developed societies, according to Giddens (1991) are based on technology and the exploitation of traditional societies that provide them with resources of food, raw materials and inexpensive labour.

Structural development

Development refers to two different processes that happen simultaneously: the improvement of socio-economic living conditions in industrialised countries and the political, economic, technological and military control of development in traditional societies (Escobar, 1995). The development of industrialised countries is based on lower levels of development in other parts of the world. According to classic economics, development has always been linked to economic growth, and subsequently it has been linked to competition rather than to cooperation. By using the same language and descriptions of people and their experience of the world we begin to see them as uniform (homogenised) rather than unique and complex. This results in the elimination of complexity and diversity of developing world peoples, so that a squatter in Mexico City, a Malaysian peasant, and a nomad in Africa all become equivalent to each other as poor and underdeveloped (Escobar, ibid.: 53–4).

For Escobar, development assumed a predetermined purpose to the extent that it proposed that the 'natives' would be reformed. This reformation would occur at the same time as reproducing and reinforcing the separation between reformers and those to be reformed by keeping alive the premise of the developing world as different and inferior, as having a limited humanity in relation to the accomplished American or European.

Mehmet (1995: 2–3) argued that mainstream economics produced flawed theories of economic development for the developing countries that resulted in distorted and biased development. He argued that Western theorists have stubbornly ignored the basic flaws in their theories, hiding these behind idealised constructions of perfect competition or rational (i.e. Western) behaviour. Overall, he argued, mainstream economists have failed to realise that underdevelopment may be causally linked to a monopoly of profits, externalities, transaction costs and other 'market failures', and above all, hidden subjective values embedded in these theories themselves.

Escobar (ibid.: 44) declared that development was – and continues to be for the most part – a top-down, ethnocentric, and technocratic approach, which treated people and cultures as abstract concepts, statistical figures to be moved up and down in the charts of 'progress'. Development was conceived not as a cultural process (with culture being viewed as a residual variable, that would disappear with the advance of modernisation) but instead as a system of more or less universally applicable technical interventions intended to deliver some 'badly needed' goods to a 'target' population.

The social and economic consequences of free-market reforms have been dramatic. In general, the primary incomes of the poor have decreased, the number of people living in poverty has increased, and social income and access to public services have decreased. Targeted interventions meant to protect the poor and vulnerable groups from the worst aspects of adjustment

failed to reach all of the poor, and seldom reached most of the poor according to a United Nations Research Institute for Social Development Seminar
(UNRISD) (Vivian, 1995).

> [In Africa] the major beneficiaries of adjustment have tended to be small
> groups of individuals with access to foreign exchange . . .
> We are witnessing peculiar types of social polarization and fragmenta-
> tion, both of which are detrimental to the social and political order upon
> which independence was built.
>
> (Bangura, quoted in Vivian, 1995)

Furthermore, a range of other social impacts is associated with free-market
reform. The UNRISD Report (Vivian, ibid.) stated that there has been a
'desocialization' of social actors, as people from community to national levels
direct their attention to coping with growing economic hardship in their
individual contexts. Inter- and intra-group conflict has increased as previous
social bonds have been disrupted and social tensions have intensified.

> In many cases, the impact of restructuring on women is especially pro-
> nounced, as the household provides the primary safety net for those
> economically displaced by restructuring. Women's reproductive work
> has thus intensified just as they are increasingly joining the labour force
> themselves.
>
> (Moser, quoted in Vivian, ibid.)

In the specific case of structural adjustment programmes, designed to comply
with the policy directives of donors and international financial institutions,
debate has raged over the causal relationship between mean restructuring and
deepening social problems. It has been argued that the latter cannot be attrib-
uted to adjustment policies, and that social problems might have been worse
had adjustment measures not been undertaken. Vivian (ibid.) claimed,
however, that it is not really necessary to address this unanswerable counter-
factual question. Adjustment measures were ostensibly meant to address
problems of poverty and inequality – to permit renewed economic growth
and development. In fact, the World Bank has said that its work must be
judged by the extent to which poverty has been alleviated. Thus, if poverty
has increased, adjustment can be said to have failed.

The psychosocial and ecological costs of full-blown industrialised societies
are harder to calculate. In terms of individual and collective morbidity and
mortality, in developed societies we are confronted with diseases and suffering hardly known to people in developing countries. While communicable
diseases still plague them, developed societies have developed a new pan-
orama of non-communicable diseases such as cancer, cardiovascular diseases,
allergies, etc. All together, the global health situation is of major concern, for

as the World Health Organization (WHO) (1999) reported, both developed and developing countries, share serious environmental health problems affecting:

- hundreds of millions of people who suffer from respiratory and other diseases caused or exacerbated by biological and chemical agents, including tobacco smoke, in the air, both indoors and outdoors;
- hundreds of millions who are exposed to unnecessary chemical and physical hazards in their home, workplace, or wider environment (including 500,000 who die and tens of millions more who are injured in road accidents each year).

Health also depends on whether people can obtain food, water, and shelter. Over 100 million people lack the income or land to meet such basic needs. Hundreds of millions suffer from undernutrition (WHO, 1992: xiii).

In addition to health problems, developing countries face a number of social, economic, cultural and political difficulties. Most of these can hardly be dealt with in short-term development programmes. Among others, they include:

- health care system,
- educational system,
- unemployment and under-employment,
- inter- and intra-country migration,
- rapid urbanisation,
- public and private transport,
- adequate housing,
- water and sanitation facilities,
- solid waste disposal,
- energy supply,
- food supply,
- population growth,
- environmental pollution.

Even more important is the awareness that local events and personal actions have become heavily dependent on developments and decisions that have their origin in other parts of the world. At the same time decisions and choices that we make here and now have a serious impact on the life chances of people living far away – in space and time. For example, each and everyone's adherence to upholding the standards of production and consumption of Western societies, not only reinforces the unequal distribution of material welfare and life chances between the rich and poor countries of the world, but also contributes to the continuing exploitation of natural resources that endangers the life and future of coming generations.

People were always insecure, but now they are being threatened on a global scale by the risks of pollution and the poisoning of food and water, and the impact of desertification, soil erosion and deforestation all of which ultimately threaten health. People's insecurity is also increasingly bound up in the risks of becoming unemployed, and of being deprived of social and physical security. This is the outcome of a worldwide dominance of social institutions that lessen the daily experiences and ethical questions that exceed the limits of their internal criteria and logic. Needs, desires and imaginations that 'escape' their logic are excluded, become objects of discipline, or are suppressed. They are seldom allowed to cause public debates about unforeseen consequences, nor about the ethical dilemmas of modern institutional ways to handle nature (including childbirth), to produce economic growth, or to control the victims of social and economic deprivation.

Public health: public trust

The 'let's all go jogging', 'stop smoking' and 'eat brown bread' type of health promotion campaigns have failed to reduce the health inequalities experienced by people subjected to modern-day poverty. Individualising the problem and the solution only damages the moral and spiritual health of the nation.

> Modern day poverty is a worse killer than smoking – and it is also passive. That is why people in my community (i.e. Glasgow) are convinced that as much passion must be applied to stubbing out poverty as is being applied to stubbing out smoking. We need homes that are fit to live in and incomes or benefits that prevent us from having to choose between heating and eating.
>
> (McCormack 1994: 10)

Cathy McCormack argued that health promotion should be concerned with living conditions because her own living conditions were not on an acceptable level for health. She argued that health promotion campaigns aimed at the individual do not make sense in the absence of adequate living conditions for human beings.

Health as defined by the WHO comprises physical, mental and social wellbeing, as an expression of trust in the present and in the future. Health is both a universal and a specific indicator for people's experience of the quality of their environment and the embedded quality of social relations they share.

Of course, wellbeing cannot be thought of without referring to trust. If people cannot have trust in themselves, they feel insecure. If they cannot trust in their neighbours, they feel insecure and threatened. If they cannot have trust in the sustainability of the environment, they lose perspective on their lives and the lives of our children and future generations. If they cannot have trust in the government, they feel alienated and excluded from the decision-making regarding their future. Trust is a key category for understanding the construction of societies (Layder, 1997, Putnam, 2002, Wilkinson, 2001). Without trust, societies would tend to be a conglomeration of individuals, more or less ordered to certain interest groups, pursuing their particular interests in competing against each other for the control of resources.

The societal development of industrialised countries, in my view, with which Cosio-Zavala and Gastineau (1997) would sympathise, has led to an almost total elimination of traditional values and belief-systems and the roles and functions of their respective institutions. Economic and technological development has simultaneously replaced traditional social systems. Traditions seem to have lost their meanings and functions for societal systems based on the individualisation of social relations in all social sectors and areas. Traditional systems of rationality appear to have been replaced with the rationality of technology. Traditional systems of inter-generational families have, by and large, been replaced with the two-generation family, although a growing proportion of the population lives alone or in single parent families. Modern societies, therefore, have become post-traditional societies in the sense that they have broken with traditions to a large extent.

Self-realisation and self-sufficiency have now become an overall ideal of human life in modern societies and are the core criteria of success (Romanyshyn and Whalen 1987). Human potential has to be developed to the fullest extent by each individual. In developed societies there is no escape from good advice about how human potential can be achieved (see Horton, 1971). People are subjected to institutions and agencies, which provide an overload of information and advice, resulting frequently in contradictory concepts and measures for improving individual lives. Advice is provided for the selection of the 'right' schools and universities, the purchase of the 'right' clothes, the use of the 'right' language and communication skills, the 'right' foods to eat, the selection of politically correct television channels to watch, the right trust funds to invest in and how to build ecologically sound homes, where to give birth, and so on. Whatever people do, there is someone 'out there' telling them how to do it correctly, often supported by some kind of statistical evidence.

Quite apart from governmental bureaucracies regulating public and private life in terms of law and order, developed societies have developed private and public organisations and agencies to design individual life itself. This has led to the development of a considerable industry dealing with every aspect of modern day life mostly covered up by labels such as 'Do-it-yourself' or 'Self-help'. These labels are euphemisms because the professional advisers or consultants do not really intend people to improve their faculties and skills. Self-help does not mean self-determination, and it certainly does not mean self-organisation or even empowerment of individuals and groups. What the consulting industry is aiming at is gaining control over individuals and the potential risks they bear for society in terms of development, creativity, solidarity and empowerment through community organisation. The focus is on self and not on help (Romanyshyn and Whalen, ibid.). It is the self as a discrete unit that is targeted, not the self as a social human being in relation to other human beings.

The consulting industry does not deal with communities or social groups but with numbers of discrete units sometimes packaged to target audiences if the issue needs to be transmitted in a relatively short period of time. The relationship between consultant and client is not always characterised by commitment, but by commerce. As soon as people have accepted the advice, that is, as soon as the advice has become the individual's property by making it part of his/her life, the responsibilities regarding the effects of acting accordingly are his/hers. Once the individual starts to jog, the heart failure is his/hers. It takes time for the consulting industry to discover whether its advice is sound. Until then, because more and more frequently unequivocal research cannot be delivered, the risks have to be borne by the individual.

Giving advice is an integral part of social relationships because it is an expression of the commitment felt to significant others. The difference between this type of advice and the advice provided by the consulting industry lies in the quality of the relationships between them as illustrated in figure 3.1, for example.

In traditional societies, societal and social processes on the whole are worked through the whole community. In developed societies, these processes are designed by functionaries and experts and are implemented subsequently according to target audiences and target areas. Developed societies have individualised human life by disembedding individuals from their reference groups and treating them as discrete units in relation to their social functions (Giddens, 1991). Developed societies have sought to organise and impose controls on individual activities but despite the prevalence of a consulting industry, individuals have been and will be unpredictable in their response to

Social relationships:	Client relationships are:
• are generally characterised by a strong responsibility for individual action • are characterised by trust • have a long-term perspective • are necessary to build communities and societies through cohesive action • are based in the context of everyday life	• characterised by the interests of the consultants to lead people on their paths of life • characterised by efficiency • short-term and outcome oriented • designed to fix 'problems' • grounded in artificial settings of professional expertise

Figure 3.1 Quality of relationships in health care

such control mechanisms as people tend to respond according to their cultural type. This is particularly true with regard to all social areas such as education, health, intimate relationships, entertainment, recreational activities or the entire leisure sector.

When internal changes in modern societies are investigated, the rapid processes of destruction of traditional values, beliefs, roles and responsibilities, education, families and so on, are almost simultaneous with processes of construction of new ways of dealing with the effects of societal changes on a human level. New values and new rituals are superseding old are replacing old values and rituals. For Illich (1976), key among these is the medicalisation of life.

Modern societies interpret social issues as social problems that need to be dealt with by professionally trained experts. In order to assign experts to 'problem-solving', the 'problems' have to be formulated in terms of the experts' knowledge base. For example, social issues such as values, family life, education, public health or nutrition are translated into categories of sociology, psychology, social work and medicine. The public discourse about these issues is translated into an expert's discourse addressing the public. In effect, the public discourse is replaced by an expert's discourse taking place in public. The public is reduced to interest groups claiming to represent the public or at least considerable segments of the public.

In conclusion, this chapter provides a contextual underpinning for the study. In the following chapters I attempt to bring women's lives more sharply into focus in the context of globalisation and localisation. What will become apparent in the following four chapters are the dilemmas facing women in childbirth as they engage in the symbolic exchanges under the influence of globalisation and localisation.

Chapter 4

Experiences of childbirth in Africa

Adwoa's story

I would like to begin with a description of a family during a period of their lives. The first part of the story concerns a woman in a small African village. I will call her Adwoa.

Adwoa is about to give birth to her second child. Her first child, a one-year-old girl called Zindzi, is often ill. Zindzi was weaned quickly onto family foods in an effort to reduce additional expenditure on milk powders.

Adwoa's day begins before the sun rises. She must fetch the water and wood from further away each day as both become scarcer. Returning home near dawn, she awakens her husband and daughter and prepares the first sparse meal of the day. There is barely enough to feed her husband and child and after they have eaten, she feeds herself and her unborn child with what remains.

Firewood and water are the most important natural resources in the lives of people in Malawi. A large proportion of Malawian households (78.5 per cent) rely on the firewood they collect as the main source of cooking fuel (87.1 per cent for rural households). An average of 6.6 hours per week is spent on collecting firewood and a further 8.7 hours on water collection. The wealthier households spend less time on these collections since they can buy firewood or hire someone to collect it for them. Apart from the possible negative effects on health and educational attainment, the time and effort spent on these activities can affect agricultural productivity and other economic activities. Urban households are more likely to acquire their drinking water from a piped water supply whether public or private (69.4 per cent). While the poorest households in rural areas acquire drinking water mainly from public sources whether protected (53.7 per cent protected wells and public taps) or unprotected (rivers, lakes and unprotected wells 38.6 per cent). Only 0.2 per cent of rural Malawian's have their own taps for their main water supply (Relative Poverty Profile of Malawi for 1998 (2001).

There are strong contrasts between urban and rural households. The most significant source of food for rural households is that which they grow in their own fields. The daily calorific value per person of food consumed is between 1,126 (rural poorest) and 2,773 (rural wealthiest). For the urban poorest the calorific value of food consumed ranges between 1,129 (poorest) and 1,995 (wealthiest). There is a dominance of cereals for the poorest households in rural areas and an increasing consumption of meat with increasing wealth (Relative Poverty Profile of Malawi for 1998 (2001).

Before Adwoa and her husband set off to work in the field, they leave their daughter with a neighbour, Rose, who is ten years old. Adwoa would like to go to the clinic to receive the care she had heard about from her friends for her unborn child, but there is simply no time. She knows she must work in order for her family to survive the season.

While in the field, she begins to feel sharp pains. Consistently, every two to three minutes, they take her breath away. Adwoa tries to ignore this interruption and continues to work alongside her husband, bent over, tilling the soil in the heat of the sun. Her own body in the process of childbirth eventually overtakes her. She cries out for her husband to fetch the local midwife. She makes her way to a nearby tree knowing that the journey home is too great. Alone, she begins active labour. The traditional midwife reaches her as the infant's head is crowning. As she hears the cry of her newborn son her first thought is 'I am alive'. Death is a constant reality for every woman in her village – for every woman in Africa.

More than half a million women die in pregnancy and childbirth every year and of these deaths, 150,000 occur in Africa. The status of women varies all over the world and nowhere do they enjoy equal status with men, but in the least developed countries, crushing poverty overlaid with long-standing patterns of discrimination create living conditions for women which are unimaginable to women in the developed world. Adjustment policies, particularly those related to financial liberation, have given a major boost to the process of globalisation. Again, evidence of the impact of globalisation on health and equity is limited, despite our knowledge that the world distribution of income has increased the gap between the world's richest 20 per cent and the world's poorest 80 per cent (Wade, 2001). Simultaneously inequality within countries has increased over the past twenty years (Cornia, 1999), resulting from:

1 trade liberalisation, which has tended to assist the import of high-tech equipment and thus privilege skilled workers;
2 financial liberalisation, which has tended to increase financial returns to capital relative to financial returns to labour;

3   inept privatisation and decollectivisation processes, which have seen assets owned by the public turned over to the private sector.

The world's poorest women are not merely poor. They live on the edge of subsistence. They are economically dependent and vulnerable, legally and politically powerless. As wives and mothers they are caught in a life cycle that begins with early marriage and too often ends with death in childbirth (Population Crisis Committee, 1988).

Adwoa's son entered a world of poverty and immediately faced the risk of dying. According to the World Health Organization (1996), an estimated 8 million perinatal deaths occur globally every year. Each year, more than 11 million children die from the effects of disease and inadequate nutrition. In Africa, more than one in five children die before they reach their fifth birthday. Many of the children who survive were unable to grow and develop to their full potential (WHO/CHD 97.12).

Adwoa is one of the fortunate ones. Her husband insists that she return home with their son to rest. He will stay at work. Tomorrow, Adwoa and her husband will return to tilling the field side by side. The newborn, Benjamin, will be with them, on his mother's back, as they work under the hot sun. Zindzi will learn to share her mother's time and attention.

The family's daily routine continues and Rose is enlisted to spend more time with Zindzi. Weakened, Zindzi is one of the first in her village to succumb to an outbreak of diarrhoea and vomiting. Adwoa seeks help from local healers, but her daughter's condition does not improve. A community health worker urges the family to take their daughter to the district hospital. Carried in her father's arms for 10 kilometres and followed by her mother and infant brother, Zindzi struggles to hang onto life. Her young body does not have the physical resources to fight the infection. She has been malnourished her entire life. She dies less than an hour after reaching the hospital. Adwoa walks home alongside her husband carrying their son on her back to face the work that was left unattended.

Years pass and Benjamin has grown into a healthy six-year-old. There is talk in the village that a school might be built. Adwoa has had three more failed pregnancies. Rose, the neighbour girl, has grown into a beautiful adolescent. At sixteen her parents were searching for a suitable husband for her. When her parents talk of marriage she only giggles. After working all day, she would rather spend her free time with her girl friends. With them she can still dream, play and hope. It is a dream or a hope that her life might be different to Adwoa's.

Rose must accept her chosen husband even though she does not know him as he is from another village. She enters marriage and leaves behind her girlish dreams, her friends and her family. Her husband is unwell and thin. Most days she must double her efforts in the fields because he is unable to work. Rose does not complain, for although he has never hit her, she knows it is possible.

(Adwoa, Ghana, 1991)

Women in premodern Ghanaian and Malawian society were seen as bearers of children, farmers and retailers of fish and other farm produce. Within the traditional sphere of Ghanaian society, the childbearing ability of women was explained as the means by which lineage ancestors were allowed to be reborn. Barrenness was, therefore, considered the greatest misfortune. In pre-colonial times, polygamy was encouraged, especially for wealthy men as a means of procreating additional labour. In patrilineal society, dowry received from marrying off daughters was also a traditional means for fathers to accumulate additional wealth. Given the male dominance in traditional society, a female's ability to reproduce was the most important means by which women ensured social and economic security for themselves, especially if they bore male children.

Oppong and Abu (1987) recorded field interviews in Ghana that confirmed this traditional view of procreation. The authors concluded that about 60 per cent of women in the country preferred to have large families of five or more children. The largest number of children per woman was found in the rural areas where the traditional concept of family was strongest. Uneducated urban women also had large families while educated and employed urban women had fewer children (see Ghana Demographic Survey, 1998).

Rose's story

As the months pass Rose finds that she is experiencing morning sickness and notices that her abdomen has enlarged. She is afraid and embarrassed. She goes to Adwoa for advice. She is gently encouraged and told what to expect during her pregnancy, but since she is often working in the fields for herself, her husband and his family, she gains little weight and feels weak.

Often women embark upon pregnancy too early and in poor health suffer endemic diseases such as malaria, tuberculosis or HIV/AIDS. They are often anaemic and many have stunted growth as a result of childhood malnutrition. Early marriage limits educational and economic opportunities and often leads to early pregnancy.

At the encouragement of Adwoa, Rose finds time to attend the clinic for one pre-natal visit. It is late in the pregnancy and she is advised to come to the clinic to deliver. She listens, but worries she will not be able to afford the cost or the time away from her husband who is now bedridden and dying.

Her husband dies before the child is born. His family offer little support and Rose is more isolated than ever. She returns to her family home and when her contractions start she makes her way to the clinic. She has an intense fear that she will also die and that her baby will be orphaned. Her labour is long and difficult. Eventually a baby girl is delivered with forceps. Mother and baby stay at the clinic for several days. Before she departs, a nurse at the clinic informs her that she, and most likely her baby, is HIV-positive.

Rose returns home and is taken in by Adwoa. She and her newborn are cared for, but she continues to deteriorate quickly. Her ability to care for her newborn becomes less and less each day. The little girl becomes an orphan at the age of three months.

Adwoa continues to care for Rose's little girl, Esi, with all the uncertainties at hand. She thinks of the daughter she lost and hopes that this child might live longer.

(Rose, Ghana, 1991)

Characterising African rural and urban society

In Ghana and Malawi the extended family system is the hub around which traditional social organisation revolves. This unilineal descent group functions under customary law. It is a corporate group with definite identity and membership that controls property, the application of social sanctions, and the practice of religious rites. Numerous varieties exist within the general framework of the lineage system. For example, in some ethnic groups, the individual's loyalty to his or her lineage overrides all other loyalties; in other groups, a person marrying into the group, though never becoming a complete member of the spouse's lineage, adopts its interests.

Among the matrilineal Akan in Ghana, members of the extended family include the man's mother, his maternal uncles and aunts, his sisters and their children, and his brothers. A man's children and those of his brother belong to the families of their respective mothers. Family members may occupy one or several houses in the same village. The wife and her children traditionally reside at their maternal house where she prepares food, usually the late evening meal, to be carried to her husband at his maternal house. Polygamy as a conjugal arrangement is declining mainly for economic reasons; but where it was practised, visitation and sleeping schedules with the husband were by arrangement.

For the patrilineal and double-descent peoples of the north of Ghana, the domestic group often consists of two or more brothers with their wives and children who usually occupy a single household with separate rooms for each wife. The largest household among the patrilineal Ewe, from Ghana's eastern coastal region, includes some or all of the sons and grandsons of one male ancestor together with their wives, children and unmarried sisters.

Irrespective of the composition of the family in either matrilineal or patrilineal societies, a senior male or headman, who might be the founding member of the family or have inherited that position, heads each family unit. He acts in council with other significant members of the family in the management of the affairs of the unit. Elderly female members of matrilineal descent groups may be consulted in the decision-making process on issues affecting the family, but often the men wield more influence.

Family elders supervise the allocation of land and function as arbitrators in domestic disputes. They also oversee naming ceremonies for infants, supervise marriages, and arrange funerals. The headman and his elders ensure the security of the family, as custodians of the political and spiritual authority of the unit. Those obligations that bind the group together also grant its members the right of inheritance, the privilege to receive capital (either in the form of cattle or fishing nets) to begin new businesses, and the guarantee of a proper funeral and burial upon death. The extended family, therefore, functions as a mutual aid society in which each member has both the obligations to help others and the right to receive assistance from it in case of need.

To ensure that such obligations and privileges are properly carried out, the family also functions as a socialisation agency. The moral and ethical instruction of children and young people is through proverbs, songs, stories, rituals, and initiations associated with rites of passage. Among the Krobo, Ga, and Akan peoples, puberty rites for girls offer important occasions for instructing young adults. These methods of communication constitute the informal mode of education in the traditional society. It is, therefore, through the family that the individual acquires recognition and social status. As a result, the general society sees the individual's actions as reflecting the moral and ethical values of the family. Debts accrued by him are assumed by the family upon the member's death and, therefore his material gains are theirs to inherit.

Land is ordinarily the property of the lineage. Family land is thought of as belonging to the ancestors or local deities and is held in trust for them. As a result, such lands are administered by the lineage elders, worked by the members of the kinship group, and inherited only by members of that group. Although sectors of such land may be leased to others for seasonal agricultural production, the land remains within the family and usually is not sold.

A network of mutual obligations also joins families to chiefs and others in the general community. Traditional elders and chiefs act for the ancestors as custodians of the community. Thus, in both patrilineal and matrilineal societies, and from the small village to the large town, the position of the chief and that of the queen mother are recognised.

The chief embodies traditional authority. Chiefs are usually selected from among the senior founders of the lineage or several lineages that are considered to be among the founders of the community or ethnic group. Chiefs have considerable executive and judicial authority. Decisions on critical issues, such as those made by family elders are based on wide-ranging discussions and consultations with representative groups from both sexes. Traditionally, legislation has not been a primary issue, for the rules of life are largely set by custom. Discussions are usually focused on the expediency of concrete actions within a framework of customary rules. Decisions, when taken by chiefs, are normally taken in council. The legitimacy of traditional authority, therefore, has usually been based on public consensus sanctioned by custom.

Although chiefs or other authority figures might come from designated families or tribes, the interest of the common people is never ignored. Where the process of selecting as well as advising chiefs is not given directly to the general population, it has often been invested in representatives of kin or local residence groups, elders or other types of council. It was such checks and balances within traditional culture that helped to balance the powers of local chiefs. It was such balances, especially among the Akan, for example, that led British anthropologist Robert Rattray (1969), to refer to the traditional political structure as a 'domestic democracy'.

In Africa, village society still forms the context in which many present-day urbanised people were born, and where some will retire and die. Until recently, the polarisation between town and village dominated African anthropology. It is crucial to realise that in the twenty-first century, even with reference to rural settings, we are not so much dealing with 'real' communities, but with rural people's increasingly problematic model of the village community. For van Binsbergen (1999) the village has become a virtual village. Throughout the twentieth century, rural populations in Africa struggled, through numerous forms of organisational, ideological and productive innovation combining local practices with outside appropriations, to reconstruct a new sense of community in an attempt to revitalise, complement or replace the collapsing village community in its viable nineteenth-century form.

If the construction of community in the rural context has been problematic, the village yet represents one of the few models of viable community among Africans today, including urbanised people (van Binsbergen, 1999). In dialogue with urban dwellers in Ghana and Malawi, the village personifies the cultural ideals of community, sharing, collectivity, history, continuity, boundaries, identity formation, family, trust, cultural alignment and spirituality.

Figure 4.1 illustrates in graphic form the contrast between traditional societies and modern societies, as perceived by participants during dialogue and is reinforced in the description of the emerging differences between the herbalist and spirit medium in figure 4.2. Modern societies are perceived to be individualistic in nature where ties between individuals are loose and people

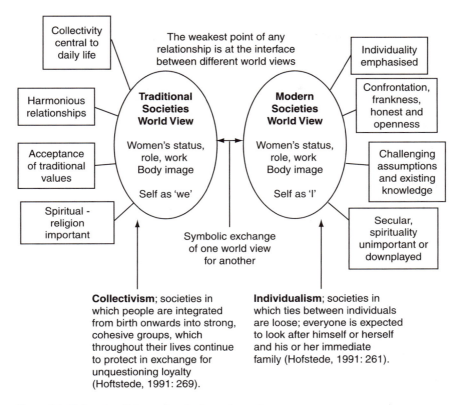

Figure 4.1 Cultural collision or symbolic exchange?

are expected to care for themselves (see also Hofstede, 1991:261). By contrast traditional societies were perceived to be concerned with collective and integrated communities producing strong cohesive groups that protect individuals throughout their lifetimes. I would argue that for development workers as for indigenous people, the weakest point of any relationship is at its interface with potentially conflicting world-views. This can result in either cultural collision in which the world-views clash and create disorienting dilemmas or in a symbolic exchange of world-views leading perhaps to a creolisation of cultural practices.

When central reproductive institutions of the old village order, including rituals of kinship, are already under great pressure from new and external alternatives in the rural environment, one would hardly expect them to survive in urban contexts (van Binsbergen, 1999). Urban life is structured, economically and in terms of social organisation, in ways that would render all symbolic and ritual reference to rural-based culture obsolete. Why do people

---

Herbalist

In his treatment of illness the herbalist relies on the knowledge he has acquired. His techniques are based on the patient's physical symptoms. While the medium immediately looks for an explanation of affliction in the woman's social relationships, the herbalist offers an explanation based on an anatomical model of the processes necessary for conception. Some of the herbalists use their interest in lorry engines to explain the dynamics of human physiology. They compare the human body to a lorry engine with its intermeshed gears and power-charged batteries (Ebin, 1982: 145). The treatment of the herbalist is directed to the patient's complaint. He is not interested in her personal relationships, either with the community or with the spirit world. Her behaviour does not affect her state of health and to this healer she does not have to explain her conduct. The herbalist's focus on the physical aspects of her affliction represents a departure from the world-view of the medium. Here then we see the separation of the body from the social being as in Western medicine.

To the herbalist, with his emphasis on learning and models of the workings of the body, childbearing is not part of an overall world-view. To him it is a different sort of problem, one, which can be seen as a discrete and isolated occurrence, and not one that reflects the core of human relationship with the social and mystical worlds.

Spirit medium

For the mediums, infertility, for example, is not seen merely as an individual malady but it becomes the focal point from which to view the client's relationship with the social and spiritual universe. Disorders of childbirth or infertility reflect a disturbance in the community; they are an index of the quality of social relations between men and the gods and are highly threatening to the community; they are a violation of the order that separates the social universe from the spirit world. The medium's treatment revolves around the transformation of the opposed concepts of dangerous and safe, heat and cool, polluted and pure. These themes are conceptualised during the treatment in the use of space between the forest and the town and in the use of red and white. As a healer, the medium is concerned not with the individual client but with the wellbeing of the community as a whole. In her view of the world, every member of the society is a catalyst to which others are vulnerable. She treats the infertile woman and at the same time protects the community from the harm she may bring. The medium seeks to control and regulate childbearing. Sexuality and childbearing are brought within the domain of culture and are integrated into an overall view of the social universe.

Figure 4.2 Symbolic exchanges amongst herbalists

pursue apparently rural forms when socially, politically and economically their lives as urbanised people are effectively divorced from the village? Staging a rural kinship ritual in town is held to restore or perpetuate a cultural orientation which has its focus in the distant village not in the intangible ideal model of community, but the actual rural residential group on the ground.

The enactment of rural rituals in urban settings is concerned with the construction of meaningful social locality out of the fragmentation of social life as experienced in urban settings in Africa and Malaysia and beyond that with the social construction of female personhood. This involves the active propagation of a specific ethnic identity among urban migrants, which serves to conceptualise an urban–rural community of interests, and assigns specific roles to villagers and urbanised people in that context (the townsmen would often feature as ethnic brokers vis-a-vis the outside world). In this way they effectively redefine the old localised and homogeneous village community into a delocalised ethnic field spanning both rural and urban structures, confronting ethnic strangers and organising those of the same ethnic identity for new tasks outside the village. In this ethnic context, the urban staging of 'traditional' rural ritual is explained as the self-evident display of ethnically distinctive symbolic production. If urbanised people stage rural kinship rituals in town it is not because they have no choice. Since rural relationships are largely reproduced through rural ritual, urbanised people stage rural-derived ritual (often with rural personnel coming in to town for the occasion) in order to ensure their ties to home and their continued benefit from rural resources: access to land, shelter, healing, historical, political and ritual office.

What I saw in Africa was neither a rejection of the old nor the complete adaptation to the modern but an amalgam of both, creating something very different from either traditional or modern – creolisation. The concept of cultural creolisation, introduced in anthropology by Hanuerz (1992), refers to the intermingling and mixing of two or more formerly discrete traditions or cultures. In an era of global mass communication and capitalism, creolisation can be identified nearly everywhere in the world but there are important differences as to the degree of exposure. Large global organisations such as the World Health Organization play a significant role in fostering the creolisation of birthing practices, for example through the training of traditional birthing attendants.

This chapter examines the symbolic exchanges (Waters, 1995) that women and midwives have experienced in the last few decades by means of narratives collected from women. The women whose stories form the basis of this chapter were all living in West and East Africa in 1991 when I was carrying out my research into Safe Motherhood Initiatives. Many changes have affected Ghanaian and Malawian women's lives over the past few decades – political insurrection, violence, poverty and so on. As the chapter unfolds some of the changes are revealed as we explore the way women's lives and childbirth are being reconstructed in Ghana and Malawi.

The reconstruction of childbirth in Africa

While visiting a small village outside Tamale in northern Ghana, I was present at a birth conducted in what I interpreted to be a traditional style. The village women sat around the hut where the woman was giving birth. They sat and told stories of their own births and the history of the birthing woman. They spoke of her birth, how the midwife had helped her into the world. They spoke of how the girl had grown and of her place within the village community. These women conveyed a message of continuity across time but contained within the confines of one place – the village. They plotted the passage of time and the changes they had seen over the years. First they explained about the advent of the training of the traditional birth attendant. The village elders had selected Akua to be trained. It was considered a great honour and there was much excitement. Then came the building of the birthing hut. All the villagers took part in creating a place for birth where the women could go to have their babies away from the family home – in peace and quiet. They told of the gathering of the women at these times to make the traditional (ritual) porridge to feed to the labouring woman to give her energy. They described a community of women that provided not only physical support through their presence but emotional and spiritual support through their united protection from harmful agents through the creation of a spiritual birthing space. From time to time the women would sing, clap and dance perhaps to convey their unity through the ritual enactment of warding off harmful spirits.

In global health development, the term traditional birth attendant (TBA) is used to refer to the diverse kinds of people who assist women in childbirth. The term TBA is commonly used in health development discourse. The abbreviation TBA stands for a complex process of translation from which it is produced and not simply for the more cumbersome generic term. TBA is an especially interesting term because it refers not to development's internal world, as do abbreviations or acronyms for agency names, but to features of the societies that development aims to change (Pigg, 1995). This abbreviation substitutes for other words in the languages of specific cultures. It is not a matter of simple abbreviation of terms in English; they foreshorten the space separating a local cultural world in which people call on certain healing specialists and an international world of health service management.

The language used by the global development authorities for talking about various indigenous healers, including midwives, has, it is argued, practical consequences. Pigg (1995) who considered that development institutions act as the locus of authoritative knowledge while devaluing other, local forms of knowledge would support my argument. Paradoxically, this devaluation of local practices occurs even as development programmes explicitly seek to work with local practitioners. Programmes for training TBAs in Ghana and Malawi offer the basis of a case study that shows how development systematically dismantles different sociocultural realities whilst taking them into account.

Mama Yawa's story

Mama Yawa is a well respected traditional midwife and spirit medium. She has had many years of experience as a midwife in her small village. Mama Yawa had undergone the government training for traditional birth attendant several years previously. In this story she is attending a refresher course for TBAs (Malawi).

Training programmes are based on a particular way of translating local African frameworks for understanding and managing birth into a generic model of birth assistance. Such translations are always problematic because the categories, values, and practices at work in one cultural context never map perfectly onto those of another. Health development initiatives that aim to spread scientific medicine and health knowledge in places where other idioms of care and healing exist face the issue of translation in their practices. Training for indigenous healers and birth attendants has been encouraged by the World Health Organization since the mid-1970s with the launching of the Safe Motherhood Initiative, as one means of achieving this goal. These training programmes seek to enhance, rather than replace them with other medical practices, by improving health service delivery through cooperation with existing indigenous systems. In the course of their implementation, however, many such programmes flounder on the ideals of 'enhancement' and 'cooperation'. In the first place, as fieldwork revealed, it is not easy to identify whom to train, or how to communicate often unfamiliar medical principles to trainees, or to introduce new practices into existing routines. Nor is it clear how indigenous practices are to be respected when the explicit goal of these programmes is to alter them, as is clearly illuminated in Mama Yawa's story.

The lesson that day began with a repetition of the main points they had covered the previous week. Sister stood in the centre of the clinic delivery room, which had been converted into a cramped lecture hall. The bed had been pushed into the middle and served as a stage on which various parts of the delivery were mimed. Sister smiled importantly round at her audience, asking for a volunteer.

One woman got up readily and, amidst murmurs of encouragement, pretended to heat some water into which she dropped some pieces of cotton. She then spread out two empty plastic sacks in front of a cardboard box that represented the labouring mother's torso. Repeating, in word and gesture, the previous lecture, she carefully wiped – from top to bottom, one side at a time, with some little pieces of cloth – round a hole cut into the side of the box, through which the baby –represented by a brown nylon stocking knotted and sewn into a baby shape – was delivered, followed by a sizeable length of plaited rope representing the umbilical cord.

'On no account should any medicine be put on the cord,' she intoned, pretending to tie the boiled cotton threads round it.

Mama Yawa didn't need to watch. She knew the sequence by heart; had even practised it in real life just the previous night. The difference was that the woman she delivered had squatted on the floor in the traditional way and was not conveniently displayed on a waist-high clinic bed; her torso had been tilted half-vertical, half-reclining – not spread-eagled on its back the way the box on the bed was. Mama Yawa had had to kneel on the cold beaten mud and bend right over to catch the first glimpse of the baby's emerging head. And then there was the mixture she had put on the cord – in direct contradiction to the clinic's teaching.

The women applauded as the first volunteer lowered a cotton sanitary towel over the gaping hole, to mark the end of her demonstration. Sister stood up again, smiling her approval, then, turning away from Mama Yawa's corner of the room, she asked if there were any questions.

Mama Yawa hesitated, intimidated by the way the nurse had so pointedly averted her body. But she caught the eye of the other nurse – who occasionally brought her own children to Mama Yawa for treatment. That nurse nodded encouragingly and Mama Yawa put up her hand.

'Yes, Mama Yawa, what is it this time?' Sister sighed, like a harassed parent addressing an irritating child. Mama Yawa asked her question. She was worried about the cord, she said. In her many years of practice – and she tried to stress the length of her experience – she had come to recognise several abnormalities of the umbilical cord, each of which could make a baby dangerously ill if it were not treated promptly by the application of some preventative potion. Everyone knew – and here she looked round at the circle of women who were listening attentively and nodding – that a baby was very susceptible to diseases carried by bad air. Bad air could enter the child by many routes, but the cord navel was one of the most vulnerable points. If they were forbidden to put anything on the cord, or give the child any medicine when it was born, how could they stop the bad air entering and the baby falling ill?

What exactly were these abnormalities of the umbilicus? Sister wanted to know, indicating by a raised eyebrow that she did not really take Mama Yawa seriously. Undeterred, Mama Yawa went on to describe in great detail certain subtle changes in skin colour and texture and in the outline of veins and arteries. She had studied these painstakingly over the years in an attempt to account for subsequent ills suffered by the children in her care. She was convinced that there was a pattern. But she failed to convince Sister, however, who stood and smiled indulgently. 'All the symptoms you describe are perfectly normal,' she pronounced kindly and dismissively. 'There's no need to treat them at all.' Mama Yawa kept standing for a while, wanting to continue the discussion, but Sister ignored her and went on to repeat her warnings about cord hygiene and eventually Mama Yawa sat down again.

The conflict raged in Mama Yawa's mind between the demands of her traditional understanding as a spirit medium and the newer demands of a changing culture and the demands of her TBA training in particular.

(Mama Yawa, Malawi, November 1991)

Such is the experience of many TBAs interviewed in Ghana and Malawi. Stories told by midwives in Malaysia also confirmed this dilemma for the TBA as was seen in the story about Azizah, where the TBA, Mek Limah was loath to undertake her traditional role in the presence of the professional midwife. These conflicts were not confined to untrained midwives either. I also found that such conflicts were experienced by professionally trained nurse-midwives in all the case study countries where they had acquired knowledge through considerable experience that did not match the official lessons they were taught in class.

At issue in training programmes is how different knowledge systems are brought together. Brigitte Jordan ([1978] 1993) observed that training programmes for traditional midwives presented cosmopolitan obstetrics as authoritative. They rendered indigenous knowledge illegitimate and indigenous ways of knowing invisible. The lesson most effectively learned by midwives and nurses was how to present themselves to the official health care system and how to legitimate themselves by using its language.

Instead of working with indigenous knowledge and ways of knowing, the training I observed attempted to override existing knowledge and practices. Trainers worked from the implicit assumption that the midwives' knowledge was wrong or inferior to the medical knowledge being presented. Jordan, drawing on her experiences concluded that by not recognising indigenous knowledge, 'cosmopolitan obstetrics becomes cosmopolitical obstetrics, that is, a system that enforces a particular distribution of power across cultural and social divisions' (Jordan, 1993:196).

Pigg (1995) looked more deeply into the ways this power asymmetry was produced. Despite a widespread appreciation of the need to take indigenous knowledge into account, training programmes continued to serve the 'cosmopolitical' function of establishing medical obstetrics as authoritative. Jordan's insightful analysis showed how this occurred in the classroom where midwives were trained. Pigg (ibid.) considered that indigenous knowledge was rendered invisible long before trainers met midwives. Training programmes, whether in Ghana, Malawi, Malaysia, or elsewhere, are embedded in a wider discourse of health development, socioeconomic politics and global imperatives that systematically produces the authoritative relationship to local cultures.

There are three issues of translation that arise in training programmes for TBAs. First, there is the problem of identifying who should be recipients of training. For example, in Ghana it became apparent that despite the diverse range of practitioners including private midwives, TBAs and government midwives, women in childbirth were seeking alternative sources of assistance. One private midwife reported that she believed that women were going to the spiritualist church for delivery. It became clear that there was a group of people who had not been identified for TBA training but who were practising.

Second, there is the problem of modifying medical messages to local contexts. Third, and least apparent to development professionals themselves and virtually unexamined in applied development writing according to Pigg (ibid.), is the problem of translating a medical model that views physical processes as separated from social contexts to other conceptualizations of well-being and illness. This is illustrated further in the following section describing the changing culture among the Aowin people of Southwest Ghana as described by Victoria.

The Aowins are a matrilineal people whose political and social organisation closely resembles that of the neighbouring Asante (Busia, 1954; Fortes, 1950; Rattray, 1923). They have a hierarchical political structure in which judicial and ritual authority rests in the office of the paramount chief who carries out his official duties with the help of the other members of his court, the queen mother, the village chiefs, the court and the spirit mediums. The female mediums are responsible for mediating between the Aowins and the spirit world and it was their official duty to maintain the wellbeing of the town.

In times of crisis, for example during epidemics, drought or heavy rains, the mediums perform the communal ritual, known as the 'momome' in which they sweep the streets of the town and outline its borders in white clay. They define the boundaries between the town and the forest and in this way express the polarity between the social universe and the world of mystical power. A harmonious relationship between men and the spirits depends on the maintenance of these boundaries. The mediums also enforce certain practices such as the use of space in town, the observance of sacred days and ritual prohibitions that form the pattern of everyday life.

In addition to their official role, the mediums also act as individual practitioners and are asked for their diagnosis and treatment of illness and affliction. In this capacity the mediums are in competition with the male herbalists who have their own distinct view of illness. Among the most common complaints they hear are those related to childbearing and infertility.

Nowadays all the spirit mediums are women and the herbalists are men, although until about 15 years ago men, too, acted as mediums and the role of the head medium was always held by a man (see Ebin, 1982: 142). This change follows a pattern seen in other roles as well. Men generally receive an education that qualifies them for better jobs. They can, therefore, abandon some of their former positions in favour of those that bring them greater income and prestige. Older women, who are generally illiterate, have access to a comparatively narrower range of occupations but they can now begin to move into the positions abandoned by men. It appears also that the restrictions imposed on the medium's personal life, as well as their official responsibilities, has less appeal for men than previously.

Men do act as healers, however, and claim to have access to mystical power, but with the important difference that they do not act as mediums of the spirits. In contrast to the roles of mediums, herbalists can practise their profession as it suits them. They are not under the authority of the chief and are not obliged, as mediums are, to use their mystical powers to protect the community. In other words, the spirit medium is concerned mainly for community healing whilst the herbalist, adopting a modernist approach is solely concerned with specialisation, individualisation, and technical skills. It is interesting to note, however, that for many herbalists, both rationality and magic coexist.

The spirit mediums, in their interpretation of misfortune, emphasise harmonious social relationships. The tension and hostility between two individuals can threaten the wellbeing of the entire community. Often the mediums will act as informal adjudicators and will intervene to give their opinions in cases of dispute. For a woman who is experiencing reproductive complications, her social relationships are a central issue in the diagnosis of her complaint. (Just as women in Malaysia, as identified in the story about Azizah, the woman must reconcile her relationships with her kin and neighbours as well as her husband). The medium organises the reconciliation and calls upon them to attend this final stage of the woman's treatment. After the purification has been performed and the woman is dressed in white they all share in a ceremonial meal.

The medium's treatment is directed towards maintaining the fabric of social life (see Ebin, 1982: 153). In her view of the world, good health depends on good behaviour. She attempts to regulate the quality of life within the town, she urges good social relations and cohesive kin ties and upholds a certain order in community life which is manifested in the use of space and in maintaining the boundaries between states of purity and pollution.

Unlike the mediums, herbalists are not part of the political hierarchy and are not under the jurisdiction of a superior. While the mediums emphasise the conservative values associated with political authority and the traditional standards of behaviour, herbalists make use of their Western education and exposure to Western ways. Some are well educated by local standards and speak English. On the whole, these men form a prosperous group: some are cocoa farmers, mechanics, school teachers and craftsmen. For all these men Western thought has played some part in their healing techniques and they augment their traditional remedies with the terms and concepts they have learned from school science books. The herbalist spends his time learning the properties of leaves and the appropriate remedies for specific afflictions. Even after the apprenticeship has ended he continues to learn new remedies. The herbalists trade such knowledge with each other and sometimes travel great distances, to acquire new and, they hope, more powerful healing remedies and charms with magical powers. The acquisition of this sort of knowledge is essential to attracting new clients and forms a basis of a herbalist's prestige. They energetically collect new formulas and recipes that are quickly discarded in favour of new and more sensational cures.

(Victoria, Ghana, 1991)

From these descriptions we begin to see the symbolic exchanges being made by the herbalists who are appropriating elements of modernity into their everyday lives and practice. This manifests itself in pseudo-scientific approaches and specialisation, in obsolescence of knowledge and in forming 'expert' communities with those who are likewise specialised. Mobility is also important as they move around the country collecting recipes and sharing knowledge. The women encountered during fieldwork were much less mobile. It would be a short step to picture these herbalists in a Western setting, attending conferences and reading the latest journals. Additionally, there is a sense of professionalisation emerging from this description. Furthermore, we are beginning to see the 'body as machine' metaphor creep into their practices.

The following account illustrates for me the diverging experiences of midwives and medical men. On a crude level one could equate the experience of the spirit mediums and the herbalists with the historical and continuing diverging experiences, world views and practices of midwives and doctors all over the world.

A major force for symbolic exchange seems to be the westernisation of thought and the subsequent implications for practice. The education and language of the herbalists seems to be implicated in their separation from their cultural worldview and practices. From my fieldwork there is clear evidence of an increasing westernisation of traditional TBA and childbirth practices, but using a set of images that may have been true fifteen years ago, but has since changed in most industrialised countries in the West. The diffusion of innovation that accounts for the new practices being introduced for TBAs and herbalists alike, seem also to not only appropriate the new but incorporate the old ways. This incorporation of new ideas into traditional beliefs appears to lead to an entirely new form of practice. This was clearly the case for the herbalists who incorporated their new learning into traditional beliefs about the body and conception but juxtaposed these with the new models of the body as machine, and the new concepts of individualism (see Keddie, 1980, for discussion on ideology of individualism).

Penetrating the village: the extension of Western ideology in the practices of traditional midwives

The modern themes of separation, measurement, surveillance, movement in labour and record keeping were observed even among the traditional midwives in Africa evidenced in the following vignette from my field notes.

Madam Nancy's story as translated by Victoria

Madam Nancy is a fifty-year-old TBA in Gondanu, a small village near Hohoe. She had been in practice for 14 years and her grandmother was a TBA. Nancy is the only TBA in the area and has a population of 4,000 people to serve. Nancy is now training her eldest daughter. She had formerly delivered women in their homes but since her training, the villages have built her a birthing hut.

I visited Nancy on a day when several women were in labour. A young woman of about twenty was pacing the room. Nancy just sat quietly watching her. She told me that she could assess the stage of labour from the way the woman was breathing and moving. Later Nancy told me that she did perform vaginal examinations to assess progress in labour. When the woman was about to deliver, Nancy took her into the birthing room and encouraged her to lie on her back on the platform built especially for the purpose of delivery.

Following delivery, Nancy completed her register of births and gave the mother a mini birth certificate which she could then take along with the baby weighing card, to the official registrar of births and deaths. After delivery, the newly delivered mother would stay with Nancy for 24 hours.

I asked Nancy about any complications she may have encountered. She informed me that she recently referred a woman with a transverse lie for caesarean section and that in the same week she detected a ruptured uterus on vaginal examination. The latter woman presented late in the first stage of labour and Nancy referred her directly to hospital.

The use of herbs was fundamental to Nancy's practice, although she would not divulge which herbs she used. This information was jealously guarded and only passed on from mother to daughter. She did tell me that she generally used herbs for perineal softening, retained placenta, postpartum haemorrhage and cord care.

Nancy's level of knowledge and experience was indeed impressive from a modern perspective. It was significant that she had abandoned traditional positions for birth currently becoming increasingly popular in Britain, in favour of an approach research has been shown to be detrimental to the health of mother and baby. Moreover, she had exchanged traditional practices for Western symbolic rituals such as vaginal examinations, and record keeping, which is mainly concerned with the concept of surveillance and control.

(Victoria, Hohoe, Ghana, 1991)

Modern rituals and childbirth practices: ritual confusion

Flora and Yaa's story

The contrast in the next story is sharp in relation to the story of Yaa and her midwife, Flora. Flora was a midwife who had trained in the UK before returning to Ghana to be posted to one of the two major teaching hospitals. She trained and worked in a large urban centre in England returning home 20 years previously and had learned a great deal about pregnancy and labour care during her training. The hospital had a team of doctors and comparatively well-equipped delivery wards. Yaa was a young woman who had moved from the rural area to live and work in the city (Ghana, 1991).

Yaa was admitted to the hospital after waiting for several days under a tree outside. She was determined to give birth in hospital. The delivery room was very crowded. Several women were in labour and two of them were giving birth as Yaa was wheeled in. There was no spare bed so she was left on the trolley. Later, as I was 'doing the rounds' with the obstetric team and I saw Yaa in one corner of the large room, a midwife was about to deliver her baby. The midwife was shrouded in green theatre gowns, gloves on her hands and a hat. A mask almost totally concealed her face. She was mumbling something to Yaa. She grunted in response and began to push – otherwise she was silent. The baby's head appeared. This happened in full sight of everyone present. There was no apparent concept of privacy. Moreover, neither I nor the doctors and other visitors were gowned in theatre attire as we wandered through the delivery suite.

Childbirth in the hospital context had truly become a public spectacle. Yaa was lying on her back with no pillows for support. The emergence of the baby was witnessed by all present. The following day, Yaa, expressed her pleasure in having had her baby the modern way. Only peasants squat and only peasants had their babies at home. When I discussed the delivery with Flora, she expressed satisfaction that Yaa had survived.

(Flora and Yaa, Ghana, 1991)

One of the key features of modern birth practices observed during fieldwork in Ghana and Malawi was the growing acceptance and desire for hospital birth where there was increasing standardisation of practices and this was confirmed during focus group meetings of senior midwives (1991). For example, on entering the hospital, birthing women were separated from their attendants; their clothes removed and ritual vaginal examinations among other measurements of her bodily functions were performed. In no cases in hospital births did I see women supported by either their husbands or female friends or relatives. The labour wards were much too busy and there was, at that time, still a belief that childbirth was women's business, except among the more 'modern' middle-class wealthy families who could afford private maternity care.

As the moment of birth approached there was an intensification of activities performed around the woman. In two hospitals I observed women labouring in the antenatal ward who, once ready to deliver, were transferred to a delivery room. The midwife or doctor routinely placed women on their backs to allow greater access; sometimes the woman was placed in the lithotomy position, covered with sterile towels and washed down with antiseptics. After the birth the baby was handed to the mother. Meanwhile she was given an injection to make her uterus contract and then her placenta was routinely extracted. If an episiotomy had been performed, it was sutured and finally the woman and her baby were cleaned up and transferred to a hospital bed and cot.

All of these activities have ritual purposes in modern society and for the object of brevity, I will only focus on two rituals for discussion. The first ritual concerns the replacement of the woman's own clothes with a hospital gown. This ritual effectively communicates the message that she is no longer autonomous, but dependent on the institution. The gown indicates the woman's liminal status (Turner, 1969: 95).

> Liminal entities, such as neophytes in initiation or puberty rites, may be represented as possessing nothing. They may wear only a strip of clothing, or even go naked, to demonstrate that as liminal beings they have no status, property, insignia, secular clothing indicating rank or role. Their behaviour is normally passive or humble; they must obey their instructors implicitly, and accept arbitrary punishment without complaint. It is as though they are being reduced or ground down to a uniform condition to be fashioned anew.
>
> (ibid.)

The gown begins a powerful process of the symbolic inversion of the most private region of the woman's body to the most public. Its openness (at the back) intensifies the message of the woman's loss of autonomy for not only does it expose intimate body parts to institutional handling and control, it also prevents her from simply walking around. The gown labels the woman as belonging to the institution (Goffman, 1961). This ritual also intensifies the strange-making process and the further breakdown of the initiate's category system.

In Africa, hospital gowns are comparatively rare items since the institution may not have the finances to provide all women with gowns. The women observed in hospital settings tended to wear their own cloths wrapped around them. These however were precarious since beneath them the women were naked and the doctors would frequently simply draw the cloth up or open without asking permission, to examine the women. The absence of seeking consent reinforced the message that the women belonged to the institutions and could be intimately touched and controlled at any time. The women observed were indeed passive and accepting of any procedure performed upon them. They had been reduced to a uniform, almost invisible, entity to be recreated in the medical image.

In the case of the second ritual, pain relief, there seems to be a fundamental assumption in Western culture that pain is bad. As a microcosm of society's culture in the condensed world of childbirth, Western cultural values stand out in sharp relief, where the medical fraternity constantly seeks to demonstrate the negative value of pain. Pain reminds us of our basic human weaknesses, and like childbirth, it reminds us of our relationship to and dependence on nature. Since modern medicine operates from the basis of the body as machine metaphor, and machines do not feel pain, it is hardly surprising that medical practitioners feel uncomfortable with women in childbirth experiencing pain, which presents a challenge to the technocratic model. Birth without pain removes half of that threat bringing us closer to the long-term goal of technological transcendence. Analgesia administered to women intensifies the message that their bodies are machines by adding a clear statement, in the case of epidurals, that their bodies as machines can operate without them. This message would not have been possible without our cultural notion of the separation of the mind and body – a basic tenet of the scientific-technocratic model. This is a model that is being globalised. In developing countries, however, as previously stated, such a model may well have long-term consequences for women who may receive and accept the model, but are unable to afford this type of care, or the drugs may well be unavailable in the hospital. In some countries the only medication available for pain relief is aspirin.

Conclusion

This chapter placed the stories of women in the foreground to illustrate their experiences as they go about their daily lives. The stories demonstrated that childbirth is being culturally transformed in Africa through the process of symbolic exchanges of childbirth rituals, into a medically dominated initiatory rite of passage through which birthing women are taught about the superiority, the necessity, and the 'essential' nature of the relationship between science, technology, patriarchy and institutions. I attempted to demonstrate how this socialisation into modern society's collective core value system is accomplished partly through obstetric procedures and partly through Western educational ideologies. The rituals of hospital birth are not only exhibited in hospital facilities but are being replicated in every village where government-trained traditional birth attendants (TBAs) practise – notions of sterility, dorsal position for delivery, examination, recorded and timed births and so on are being embedded. I presented illustrations of how these procedures work to map the technocratic model of reality which underlies modern society's core value systems onto the birthing women's perceptions of her childbirth experience, with the goal of achieving complete conceptual fusion between this technocratic model and the belief systems of birthing women.

The key symbolic exchanges observed in Ghana and Malawi that have implications for a universal midwifery curriculum were centrally concerned with:

- collective versus individual: imagined communities?
- technological ideology – as a metaphor for practice in the absence of technology;
- new rituals for old;
- measurement – positivism;
- surveillance and control;
- specialisation.

In this chapter I have applied an eclectic model derived from sociology to women in childbirth which interprets this process as a rite of passage. In so doing, I have sought to illuminate the underlying cultural significance of symbolic exchanges in childbirth, concerned mainly with the globalisation of symbols and signs of modernity, and its uses. I argued that childbirth is a rite of passage of tremendous cognitive significance for women across the globe; that messages conveyed by the rituals of hospital birth both reflect and reinforce the core values of modern societies originating in the West (that is the USA and Europe). The messages conveyed by antenatal care and the rituals of hospital birth both reflect and reinforce the core values of modern society (principally American). These rituals transform women in childbirth in ways that reflect their orientation to those core values and to the technocratic belief system that underlies them.

In Africa, these things are not entirely overt but what is being transmitted are the symbols and signs of this belief system although the actual physical tools are lacking. These messages are conveyed in conversations, in shared ideologies, in imagined communities. These symbols are promoted by such agencies as the World Bank and WHO, IMF and so on. They are conveyed in the imperatives placed on governments to conform to global 'standards' of health care, the models for this standard care being those exemplified in American medical facilities. Africa cannot aspire to that level of care, however, so all they are left with are the ideologies and not the wherewithal to make a difference in their system. The application of time and measurement, of rules and policies that control birth does not cost money, so we are left with a high technology ideology without the high technology equipment – the Emperor's new clothes.

The role of women in relation to risk, with special emphasis on the state of the environment and development is now recognised in some areas but still does not feature as the prime focus of many programmes for the major governmental or non-governmental aid agencies. It is an issue that is highly important, not only for the environment and development, but also for the health and wellbeing of women themselves. In developing countries, many women's relationships with the environment are vital to their daily lives, for example, the provision of water, fuel, food and other basic needs. These women do not only bear the brunt of environmental degradation, but also play a crucial role in environmental management. Women everywhere are influencing the environmental debate in a numbers of ways – as consumers, as educators, as campaigners and communicators.

In the next chapter we travel to a country in the process of rapid modernisation under the influence of globalisation – Malaysia. There we will explore the experiences of women who live in a society that is undergoing rapid urbanisation, has both poverty and wealth, has high technology, is developing financial, communication and transport systems, but at the same time suffers from many of the problems of developing countries.

Chapter 5

Experiences of childbirth in Malaysia

Aminah's story

Aminah was a young woman who had moved to the city to find work. She was also keen to see and experience a way of life she had heard about from friends – a life that was very different from her own in the village.

I took a job in Kuala Lumpur, leaving my *kampong* (village) and poorly paid local jobs for a better salary in the capital city of Malaysia. Although better paid by comparison, the money I earned working in the Texas Instruments factory was still very low and I had to share my sleeping quarters with three other young women. I worked on rotating shift in the factory. The conditions were harsh and my family was concerned for my health. I already had a health problem that I had consulted both traditional healers and Western medical practitioners about [*without resolution – ed.*].

My mother hoped to buy some land for growing vegetables and perhaps rubber tapping to encourage her daughters to work with her. But I, although hating my job, chose to continue working there in the hope of winning the firm's lottery with a prize of a free trip to the United States. I do return home for celebrations [life-cycle events] or for an Islamic occasion, taking a break from work to visit my family and friends [reaffirming ties with family and the traditions of our community].

(Aminah, Malaysia, 1993)

This brief glimpse of the lives of a woman and her mother in Malaysia gives a sense of the profound changes occurring in their lives but also of the continuing importance of age-old patterns of behaviour and belief. What this snapshot can only hint at is the way in which both the important transformations and the persistence of traditions are linked to the growing incorporation of Malaysian society into the international capitalist economy.

Malaysia, like many countries in the developing world, has been undergoing a process of intensive capitalist development. This entails the extension of capitalist property relationships in both agrarian and industrial sectors, a growing incorporation of people into an international division of wage-labour, and increasing dependency on a cash economy in a competitive world market. While these changes are encouraged and supported by Malaysian government policies, the new economic forces and their penetration into the local context are largely controlled by and under the direction of multinational corporations and financial institutions (Lim, 1982; McAllister, 1987: 88–93; Ong, 1983, 1987; Jomo, 1988; Scott, 1989).

Such processes induce a fundamental transformation, often rapid and abrupt, of traditional societies and cultures. In Malaysia, this affects even those sectors of the Malay ethnic groups left untouched by the earlier period of European colonialism. The current transformations most seriously affect women and thus are revealed through the changes in their lives.

Persistence and change

Neither capitalist development as it is occurring in Malaysia today, nor its effect on women, is a simple unilineal process. Instead, along with the growth of a wage-and-market economy and the new social relations and cultural conceptions this induces, there is also the persistence of traditional economic and social forms and accompanying value systems and world-views. For some parts of Malaysia, such as the Negeri Sembilan, this means particularly the continuation of matrilineal and Islamic traditions. In spite of extensive economic and social restructuring, such traditions are not being simply replaced by new forms of organisation and belief; nor are they mere 'vestiges' of a previous stage of social evolution about to disappear (McAllister, 1992: 90). Rather, both matriliny and Islam persist as vital and evolving components of people's lives and, as such, continually develop new points of accommodation and conflict with each other as well as with the increasingly dominant capitalist system.

Village women creatively adapt both economic and social practices to their new circumstances and then use these renewed traditions to meet changing needs. McAllister (ibid.: 108) suggested that the revival and elaboration of communal practices provide these women and their families with a support system that buffers them from some of the more exploitative features of the wage-and-market economy into which they are increasingly drawn. At the same time, such matrilineal forms can become undermined and distorted by their encounter with capitalist relations and values, with particular results for women's roles and gender relations. It is these contradictory dynamics of the current transformation in political economy that we must grasp to understand the choices of women in Malaysia.

McAllister (ibid.: 109) drew three conclusions from her study of the Negeri Sembilan women that she considered must be taken into account in any general model of developing world change. First was the fact that the co-existence of various aspects of the matrilineal and capitalist systems was not a static or stable situation. Rather what she saw was an active interpretation and reworking of these different forms in a process that involved both accommodation and conflict. Rather than just being maintained, aspects of the matrilineal system were frequently revived, elaborated, and extended to new situations. This also applied to the management of childbirth. Through this process, however, such 'renewed traditions' can become more fundamentally transformed, sometimes experiencing a weakening or reformulation of core meanings or principles. The rise of religious movements, especially the fundamentalist Islamic revival in Malaysia must also be taken into account. The global Islamic revival not only transformed traditional Malay Islam, it affected the surviving matrilineal systems as well. The complex dialectical nature of these multiple interactions and their implications for the overall picture of social transformation must be grasped within any analysis of the contextual relationships in Malaysia that influence the experience of women in childbirth.

Second, McAllister (ibid.: 109) urged us to recognise that this process of uneven and combined development affects different sectors of the population in different ways. Bee's story, for example, illustrates the impact of capitalist development, globalisation and modernity on women's lives alongside their continued involvement in traditional birthing practices as a buffer against new forms of exploitation and stress. Women play a significant role in the perpetuation and elaboration of these traditional forms and the survival of aspects of the matrilineal (including birthing) system had particular benefits for their lives.

Bee is an experienced midwife working among women from both the town and nearby kampongs. She qualified in Malaysia and had participated in post-qualifying programmes in America and the United Kingdom. Bee had studied extensively and had undertaken some development work with the World Health Organization. She also had experience of conducting research, and had participated as a team member for some medical research. This is one of Bee's stories that demonstrates her frustration and desire to improve maternal health care in her own country.

Azizah's story as told by Bee

Azizah sat among a group of expectant mothers patiently waiting for her number to be called. She had never missed a single appointment. She looked a picture of health.

'I'm amazed at the rate my baby grows,' she once said cheerfully, 'My mother-in-law is even more excited than I am. It's going to be her first grandchild.' She was radiant and beaming with pride. Azizah's husband worked as a clerk in a school nearby and often took time off to accompany her to the clinic. Like most first time expectant parents, they were keen participants of the health education sessions held regularly at the clinic.

This health centre which Azizah was attending was in a remote district in one of the east coast states of Peninsular Malaysia where I once worked some 14 years ago. Like all other government health centres, it offered a range of services including domiciliary midwifery services. The longest serving officer at that centre was Fatimah, a midwife who had been at the centre for more than 12 years. She was a familiar figure among the villagers. When I was first posted to this place, it was Fatimah who oriented me to this village community and introduced me to the formal and informal leaders.

Traditions die hard in this village and physical changes and modernisation appeared to have little influence on traditional values and practices. These traditional practices were evident especially in childbirth, postdelivery, confinements and childrearing practices. Not all beliefs and practices were detrimental to health though. In fact, there were those which enhanced and promoted health.

Late one night, I was called to help Fatimah who was attending to a case of home delivery. The patient was Azizah and she had already been in labour for some time when I was called in, for it appeared that Fatimah had not been successful in trying to convince the family to get Azizah to hospital. I envisaged a difficult task ahead of me. I could not believe that the patient she was dealing with was Azizah for she and Hashim, her husband, had always been very cooperative.

There were already a number of people in the house when I arrived, both men and women, some of whom I was familiar with like the headman, the traditional birth attendant (TBA), Mek Limah and Azizah's mother-in-law. From a distance I could smell the burning of incense and the smell of traditional Malay linament used for massaging. Azizah was lying on a mattress on the floor in a corner of the hall with Fatimah and the TBA attending her. Her family, especially her mother-in-law, was adamant about using traditional methods and it was apparent that she did not want hospital treatment though modern treatment in the home was acceptable.

During the course of my interactions I realised that the deep-rooted fear was actually the fear of surgical interventions. Azizah's labour had been prolonged and she was still at home. I felt a deep sense of remorse seeing her suffer excruciating pain and being denied the treatment, which was easily available. She appeared relieved to see me. After a quick and thorough assessment I called for the ambulance in readiness, although I knew that it would take time to convince her people to give consent.

The presence of pressure from the elders had caused Hashim to become rather passive. I resented that Azizah's husband did not make an effort to intervene in this crucial decision which concerned the safety of his wife and child. Caught in this situation, I realised how I had underestimated the strength of influence extended families had.

The greatest hurdle was actually the presence of a prominent 'bomoh', a traditional healer, who was called by the family for consultation and to carry out traditional treatment, as the more common practices provided up to then had failed. Religious and magical systems excluding modern medical concepts of disease had placed traditional healers on the first line of intervention. I knew that everybody present was deeply concerned about Azizah's safety and that they were doing their best to remove 'barriers' that were causing the delay in the delivery. It was a matter of perception and belief and I endeavoured to alleviate this ignorance.

Soon all drawers were opened, doors kept ajar and they went to the extent of unstitching ends of pillows that were available in the house. As time went on everyone especially the women folk were in a sort of frenzy. Azizah was asked to repent to her husband for her past 'wrong doings' and he was made to walk over her abdomen back and forth many times and a host of other things which seemed quite impertinent to me!

I desperately wanted to help this lady whose prolonged sufferings were unnecessary. I thought this was more than a health issue, it was a human issue and a woman's rights issue! Where else could I get help? I had to explore all avenues. The influential people were already there and I had to talk to them.

When the ambulance arrived, I had wished I was in control of the situation. Explaining to the ambulance team that Azizah was not ready to go was another issue. 'We have to give Azizah a chance to deliver by herself,' her mother-in-law said firmly. 'We are all here to help her.'

Slowly I began to see light at the other end of the tunnel. In the course of the event, they appreciated our anxiety and sincere desire to offer the best service available. They became more attentive to our explanations and asked a lot of questions expecting positive answers. Gradually they accepted that being given traditional and medical treatment together Azizah would be provided with the best of care. When it was time to wheel Azizah into the ambulance everyone lent a hand and we worked at top speed.

Azizah underwent a caesarean section and her baby boy was asphyxiated at birth but was well after resuscitation. A month later she was back at the health centre, this time with the baby in her arms. Seeing both mother and child well and healthy gave me a sense of satisfaction and pride.

(Bee, Kuala Lumpur, 1993)

There are a number of key points that can be drawn from this story. Bee herself identifies a number of salient issues, namely the complexities experienced by midwives in cultural situations, especially where they have to face the full blown cultural influences of the village community. For as she says, 'modernisation appeared to have little influence on traditional values and practices' in village life in Malaysia. She came to understand her deficiencies in her understanding of culture and concluded that she should not have taken Azizah and her husband's ability to control their own birth experiences for granted, finally realising how deeply rooted traditional beliefs were and how this affected their behaviour. Bee also came into conflict with her peers because of the delay in transferring Azizah to hospital. Bee clearly experienced horizontal violence (Spring and Stern, 1998) towards her because she failed to comply with hospital routines.

Pryia (1992: 67) found that whatever the religious beliefs of traditional midwives in Malaysia, the incantations they used and the spiritual help they sought often came from a much wider or older spiritual tradition. In Malaysia, however, those of a more fundamental Islamic persuasion condemned the Malay Muslim traditional midwives for such practices. This appears to be the case here.

Bee goes on to say, 'To us outside the culture, their behaviour and ways of dealing with the difficult labour had appeared strange and wrong but to the insiders it is what they have learnt through the ages as being normal and appropriate way of dealing with the problem.' Furthermore, she highlights that the different ways of tackling the situation were due to differences in beliefs and theories. The midwives' beliefs were based on current medical knowledge that made the assumption that prolonged labour is dangerous for mother and baby. This knowledge created a sense of urgency to get the labouring woman to hospital – as the only right and proper place to deal with this emergency. Azizah's kin viewed the problem as a result of supernatural forces or sorcery. In this scenario, their actions were suitable. The dichotomies encountered by midwives are considerable and the introduction of new ideas from outside the culture proves every bit as disorientating for trained midwives as for traditional attendants.

At the same time, the distortion of such traditional practices that often results from their interaction with the emerging capitalist, global medical systems had a special effect on gender roles and relationships, in this case the undermining of pre-existing situations of relative gender equality. This occurred even though traditional ideology of gender relations may have remained in force (see McAllister, 1989b).

Finally, McAllister suggested that models of change in the developing world must take account of the power relations involved in this 'balancing act' of old and new. She observed (1992: 110) that Negeri Sembilan women often used their continued involvement in matrilineal practices as a form of resistance against absorption into the wage and market system. Abu-Lughod

(1990) in an analysis of fieldwork based on Bedouin women suggested that changing forms of resistance should alert us to changing forms of power. She also warned against romanticising resistance, which often appears very creative and resilient, without noting the creation of new dimensions of power to which it is a response. Both of these points are well taken. For McAllister, the Negeri Sembilan women were not engaging in new forms of resistance; those being employed by the women were of long-standing economic and cultural practices of daily life that were being converted into vehicles of resistance. In other words, what people were doing was not so new, but why they were doing it was. The different aspects of traditional culture survived primarily as ways of providing protection from or resistance to the developing capitalist system.

This transition occurred because of the imposition of new forms of power held by employers, the state, health care workers and international financial institutions, to name just a few (Abu-Lughod, 1990). What was equally important, was whether such a transition would result in new divisions of power among the Malaysian people themselves – e.g. on the basis of gender or class. One could argue that given some of the distortions occurring in traditional practices, this might seem likely. On the other hand, everyday resistance continued through the acts of matrilineal practices that may presage another outcome, one in which the basic principles and practices helped shape the more conscious struggle for self-determination that is developing in Malaysia and throughout much of the developing world today. It is this larger 'balancing act' between the further undermining of traditional egalitarian forms or the use of such forms as effective resistance against new inequities brought about by globalisation that represents the most important power struggle in contemporary Malaysian society. Its progress and outcome will fundamentally affect the lives of women and of their communities.

The impact of modernity on Malaysian women in childbirth

Women from traditional societies are usually vague about when birth is likely to take place. In modern societies doctors are very concerned to pinpoint the expected date of delivery from which all interventions proceed thereafter if the pregnancy ends early or later than predicted. In contrast women in traditional societies had a more relaxed approach to this. They usually knew within a month or so as to when the baby might arrive and trusted to their own internal knowledge and experience of the pregnancy as to when birth would take place. In their own minds they made no distinction between the means used to ensure a successful pregnancy and those they took to ensure an easy birth, although inevitably some of the things they did focused more on birth than on pregnancy.

In modern societies the length of labour also has an expected period of time for each stage. When speaking with traditional midwives about how they assisted women in labour, it soon became apparent that what I meant by labour, being brought up in the Western ideology of labour, was rather different to their interpretation of labour. I thought of labour as occurring in three stages: the first stage when the cervix opens, the second stage, when the baby is expelled and the third stage when the placenta is delivered. The separation of labour into stages is an attempt to impose an order on it that in the minds of traditional midwives and the communities they serve, does not exist. The traditional midwives interviewed took a much more concrete view of labour. They concern themselves primarily with the delivery of the baby. The rest of labour seemed to merge imperceptibly into ordinary life and was considered far more idiosyncratic, particularly in terms of the extent to which a woman might ask for help at this time.

The traditional midwives believed that women experienced labour in as many different ways as there were women. They found it difficult to talk in generalities, instead, as Priya (1992: 64) discovered they chose to speak about individual cases and concrete situations. They told stories of different women and their families to illustrate their point – that each woman was different. Whilst there were general principles, the important factor for them was to respond to the needs of the labouring woman, which may mean that at times, they may not follow their own general principles. For them labour and birth was a time of maximum vulnerability. The type of help a woman may need was not only in relation to what was happening in her body, but how she was experiencing it and the supernatural forces that may be hindering or helping the process. The expertise of these traditional midwives lay in their ability to gather all their knowledge and skills at all levels in response to the woman's individual needs.

In many places around the world there are special ceremonies undertaken around the time of birth to ensure a safe and easy delivery. To give birth, a woman must allow her body to open and to release the child. In the West, preparations for this usually include various physical exercises whereas in traditional societies women prepare by symbolically clearing the way, a process that is often described as sympathetic magic. They avoid all thoughts and actions which have anything to do with becoming stuck or closing up in case this is transferred to their body and the child becomes stuck or their body refuses to open easily to give birth.

A very common action of this type, which was described to me, was the behaviour of pregnant women in connection with entrances and exits to houses. Malay pregnant women avoid sitting in the doorway of their house or on the steps leading up to it in case this should cause a blockage and the child finds it difficult to be born. They are also careful to go out of the house by the same door that they entered.

To enable her body to be opened easily the pregnant woman should not do anything to place herself in a situation, which implies a closing up, or the making of an obstruction. In many places the wearing of belts or necker-chiefs is discouraged to prevent knots in the umbilical cord. In Sarawak, pregnant women avoid tying things together with rattan. If this is a job that has to be done then a non-pregnant woman is asked to start the job which the pregnant woman then finishes so that possible negative consequences are neutralised.

In traditional societies, it is generally believed that women who work hard are more likely to have an easy delivery; this is not only because it keeps them physically active but because it keeps them, and therefore their baby, 'loose' so that it will be born more easily. Birth preparation in the West is much more physically based, with various breathing exercises forming a large part of what is taught in antenatal classes. The roots of modern birth preparation stem from the work and writings of Grantley Dick Read whose first book on the subject was published in 1944.

The traditional midwives I spoke with did not expect to have many difficul-ties as, in their experience, most women gave birth without problems. They were, however, confident that they would be able to deal with any complica-tions that might arise, especially when they had the assistance of their guiding spirit to whom they could turn for more powerful help. If the labour is prolonged various methods are used to entice the baby out of the womb. The midwife may instruct the husband to step over his wife's supine body three times to graphically show which gender is superior. The woman may have been unfaithful and/or strayed from her prescribed feminine role by not being passive and submissive enough. By acting out the different gender roles in this way, order and harmony is restored and the baby can be born.

In Sarawak, if labour is prolonged, two medicine men are called to perform a special ritual. One goes inside the house and the other stays outside. The one inside places a loop of cloth around the labouring woman while the one outside places a loop of cloth around his own waist with a stone in it. This is followed by a long incantation sung by the man outside. The man inside uses his psychic powers to force the baby downwards and as the child descends, the tightly tied cloth is moved downwards to prevent the baby moving back up. The one inside shouts to his companion who moves the stone downward in mimicry of the baby. This proceeds until the child is either born or until everyone becomes convinced of the fruitlessness of his or her efforts.

If these normal methods fail then the midwife calls on a more powerful person to divine what the problem is and what further measures should be taken. A *bomoh* (local medicine man) would be called to whisper to the spirits, especially the good ones, to help banish evil spirits.

Domicillary deliveries were always the responsibility of *bidan kampung* (traditional midwives) but since independence and the resulting political shift, educated young women were trained as auxiliary midwives and sent to serve in rural communities. It soon became clear that these young, educated women were coming across some strong resistance from the established traditional midwives who naturally felt threatened both in terms of livelihood as well as social status. Colson (1969) observed that the trained midwife in the village she studied never attended a birth independent of the traditional midwife but that the traditional midwife attended many births without the government midwife. This was also the case in Bee's story. Maintaining good relationships with the traditional midwife was considered important although frustrating at times.

Chen (1975) noted that during childbirth, the traditional midwife, if she was the midwife of choice, attended the delivery alone as she was perceived by the family to be willing and able to attend to all the needs of the mother during childbirth. Conversely, she noted that the villagers considered that the trained midwife only performed three of the fourteen traditional duties expected of the *bidan kampung* and that eighty per cent of mothers had to employ a traditional midwife if they wanted the remaining eleven traditional duties to be performed.

Although the trained and traditional midwives would conduct themselves with decorum, as required by Malay culture, they were covertly suspicious and resentful, treating each other as rivals rather than allies with a common objective. The *bidan kampung* should have been subordinate to the trained midwife since she had little training and her techniques were sullied by supernatural hocus-pocus according to Bee. Further the trained midwife knew that half of the mothers attending clinic would be 'stolen' by the traditional midwife for delivery. On the other hand, to the traditional midwife, the government midwife's air of superiority was insulting since she had no claims to the vast wealth of traditional knowledge about birth and life that distinguished the traditional midwife from ordinary women. Moreover, the trained midwives were always younger and thus less experienced.

Nowadays, the greater majority of women deliver in hospital under the care of doctors. To counter this trend and to incorporate the traditional midwife into the health team, new roles have been developed for each so that the midwife and *bidan kampung* can cooperate and support each other. The trained midwife, who has received at least twenty-four months of training, is supported by nursing supervisors, doctors and the hospitals, and is responsible for the actual delivery of the mother, cutting the cord and the care of the newborn. She is also able to detect and refer high-risk cases and complications to the more qualified supervisors and doctors.

Members of a focus group of senior midwives (Kuala Lumpur, Malaysia, 1994) reported that 'trained midwives do not receive instruction in the traditional duties expected by the communities they serve as part of their midwifery training.' The absence of local traditional birthing practices is evident in the government defined midwifery curriculum. The traditional midwife would be expected, for example, to provide advice and instructions concerning the antenatal taboos and behavioural avoidances that the family had to observe in order to ensure a safe delivery and a normal infant. She would be responsible for supervising the performance of precautionary measures during labour; to ritually bathe the mother; to supervise the ritual disposal of the placenta; to wash soiled linen; to provide advice and instruction concerning dietary taboos after childbirth; to supervise the 'roasting' of the body and abdomen and to provide 'heating medicines'. According to Alice – a midwife working in Kuala Lumpur, Malaysia, who participated in a focus group discussion – the traditional midwife would also be expected to perform the traditional postpartum massage of the mother's body (focus group discussion, 1994).

Government-trained midwives not only lack training and knowledge in these matters but they are also rarely inclined to provide many of these services. Neither does the trained midwife have sufficient time to stay with the family to cook and to wash for the whole household (Connie, focus group discussion, 1994). The traditional midwife, on the other hand, is the person obviously best suited to carry out most of these traditional duties. She also supports breast-feeding and she can give advice on family planning (Ong, focus group discussion, 1994). She would, in an emergency and in the absence of the trained midwife, deliver a mother and cut the cord (May, focus group discussion, 1994). The traditional midwife would also be given appropriate training to prevent harmful practices being conducted (Mahani, focus group discussion, 1994).

Chen (1975) reported that in their readjusted roles the midwives complemented each other. At the first sign of labour the *bidan kampung* is summoned, and begins to carry out all the precautionary measures traditionally expected of her. Once the second stage of labour begins, she sends for the trained midwife who then conducts the delivery, cuts the cord and bathes the baby. Throughout labour, the traditional midwife sits opposite the trained midwife and from time to time mutters a prayer or a charm to reassure the labouring woman.

Interestingly, when I was in Malaysia in 1994, the two-year training of midwives was coming to an end because it was considered that they had insufficient knowledge for effective performance of their role. The new policy was to ensure that all midwives had a nursing qualification before undertaking a midwifery programme. One obstetrician observed that the midwives had very little medical knowledge and that it was important that the training was lengthened to encompass more nursing and medical knowledge.

Rapid changes in health services have been implemented over the last two decades. District services have been decentralised and hospitals up-graded for diagnostic and management support of childbearing women. Antenatal screening has been refined and a national confidential inquiry into maternal deaths introduced. District teams have been trained in problem solving and management and health professionals retrained to improve their skills. TBAs have also been retrained as partners to the health professionals able to refer pregnant women while retaining their role in providing emotional support to the woman and her family. Skilled professionals conduct increasing numbers of deliveries and alternative birth centres have been introduced in rural and urban areas. Alongside these improvements, functional referral and emergency transport systems have been implemented with the result that maternal mortality fell from 300 per 100,000 in the 1960s to 40 per 100,000 live births in 1997. Attendance of a skilled provider at birth rose from 57 per cent in 1980 to 95 per cent in 1996 (Litsios, 1997). But what does this mean for women?

There are sharp contrasts between women's experiences of childbirth in Malaysian hospitals, as illustrated in the story in chapter one. Nurse-midwives and doctors interviewed were convinced that the safest place for birth was the hospital under the care of an obstetrician to prevent death and yet the experience for many women is perhaps less than satisfactory.

In a telephone interview with a renowned author and social anthropologist, Priya (1998), concluded that modern and traditional ideas and approaches to birth seem so very different that it is very difficult to find points of contact between traditional and Western practices. The woman in the West expects to receive medical care during her pregnancy and labour and the vast majority go to hospital to give birth. This would probably be unimportant if pregnancy and birth were viewed as normal processes but the woman's experience from antenatal care onwards would be one of seeking and finding problems and perhaps being told that she is part of a high risk group and thereby more likely to develop complications. She will either explicitly or implicitly be expected to defer to the doctor's ideas as to what is most appropriate for her and the responsibility for finding and dealing with problems will be the doctor's rather than hers.

With almost 95 per cent hospital deliveries (as reported by the Supervisor of Midwives, Ministry of Health, 1997), Malaysia has gone a long way down the road of incorporating Western medical ideals into the everyday experience of women. This might not be quite so straightforward as it at first appears.

Patricia's story

Patricia provided some insights from her own observations in Malaysia in 1997.

Malaysia is 30 years behind the times – they are conforming to things that are not done now in the UK – they think they are modern but it is vital to look at the local situation when adopting Western medicine. In the rural areas of Malaysia, like India, there are no real motorable roads. Getting a woman to hospital when in trouble is a problem – the only means of transport is by ox cart which is very slow and women usually give birth in the cart before they reach hospital. This is very embarrassing and consequently women tend to go to hospital before labour starts. Of course there is only hospital-based medicine – hospitals are in the towns – not in the villages.

Women are being regimented in a way that women were regimented 30 years ago in the UK – but more exaggerated . . . worse in many ways . . . staff are overworked – impersonal. Women are not allowed to have their families with them during labour which is against their traditions . . . this creates a conflict and it is not surprising that women end up with caesarean sections . . . there are six women labouring and giving birth in a room – this is not a private space. The labours are very managed – they love to put up drips with drugs to get them going – to hurry labour along. Care is based on doing the technical stuff properly, not on caring for women.

My interpretation of this comment was that Patricia was inferring that because of the conflict women experienced between their own culture and traditions and those of the imposed culture and rituals, a situation is created in which labour is more complex, dangerous and complicated. That is, the consequences of a cultural clash for women may result in a more dangerous labour, which may increase rather than decrease morbidity.

In Kuala Lumpur I went to a public hospital for a Rhesus test for my last baby. Given that this was exotic and unusual – the Malaysians don't have a Rhesus problem – I was to see the British doctor. Whilst at the hospital, I saw these women lining the corridors, alone – no family around them. A friend of mine is married to an obstetrician who works in the Chinese hospital in KL. She is very pro natural childbirth, etc., and he has set up a birthing room but no-one uses it, except perhaps some foreign women. If I had been going to give birth in hospital that is where I would have had my baby. But the Chinese did not want this. They pay more for anaesthesia than for acupuncture, which is available in the birthing room. More and more Chinese women are requesting caesarean sections (C/S), and my friend's husband says he turns down two or more per month. He will not perform C/S unless there is a reason but he knows his colleagues do. A C/S costs around $2000. Doctors make more money by performing them rather than allowing vaginal birth.

It seems that when medicine is taken into another country it gets corrupted according to the local situation. Ideas are taken and distorted. This half way place creates conflict. Another example is that mothers are more likely to give their babies processed foods than the locally available foods. It seems ridiculous to me that they will give dried bananas from a packet when they can get fresh bananas from the market practically free. There is something very strange about the way in which Western knowledge and actions are adapted in the local setting.

Take the ideas about the body and the way it works. The Chinese have a thing about hot and cold foods. Pregnancy is considered a hot state therefore women will not take vitamins during pregnancy because they are also hot. There is a superimposition of Western ideas onto traditional ideas that can cause real problems. Some of the beliefs generated can be really bad for mother and baby. How new ideas from other cultures and situations are interpreted is really important. Take the village health workers – they are taught to weigh pregnant women, take their BPs and test urine but they don't look at the results nor do they interpret them or realise the implications. In a village in Malaysia all the pregnant women were weighed but there was something wrong with the scales since all the women weighed the same – not only from one visit to the next, but as each other. The village worker weighed them religiously but failed to recognise the implications of what was happening. It takes on an element of magic – of ritual – if we do this then the baby will be all right.

When a doctor visited a village health centre, he examined a woman and found that the baby was in a transverse lie. When he pointed this out and asked how long this had been the case, the village health worker said yes, she had noticed but had said nothing, assuming the baby would turn. This was nearing the due date. Yes the baby might well turn but should the woman go into labour, and the lie remain transverse, then no-one would know anything about it because the health worker failed to see the significance. She had ritually examined the woman but did not connect that to the importance of taking action. Just doing the examination in her eyes and maybe that of the woman was enough to ensure that everything would be all right. There is an element of that in the West too. Women assume that just by having all the tests the baby will be all right.

In another incident a further aspect of modern ritual was highlighted. When women are pregnant they are given an injection. They go to a government clinic. But when I asked what this injection was for they could not tell me other than to say that it made them strong. It took me ages to find out that this injection was tetanus but the myth had been built up that this was good and yes it was, but not for the reasons they believed it to be. The women would only have the injection on the third, fifth or seventh month because those are considered the luckier months of pregnancy. This overlay of Western medicine and traditional beliefs is very interesting. The injection had been worked into a ritual process – to guarantee a good birth and healthy baby.

(Patricia, Malaysia, 1997)

In traditional societies, pregnancy and birth are normal processes central to the life and identity of a woman. In the main a pregnant woman receives advice and care from female relatives and friends and has access to the help of a more experienced traditional midwife or other traditional specialist should she need it. She protects herself not only from physical harm with various rituals but also spiritually by harnessing positive forces to protect her and her baby. The woman is in control of the process and through this control she has a measure of security that is bolstered by centuries of tradition. In these modern times, women's lives, even in rural areas, are changing but they may be unwilling to entirely give up their traditions and health services are beginning to take account of this.

Conclusion

The brief vignettes from the lives of a few women in this chapter are an attempt to provide a sense of the profound changes occurring in Malaysia and also of the continuing importance of age-old patterns of behaviour and belief. What these snapshots can only hint at is the way in which both the important transformations and the persistence of traditions are linked to the growing incorporation of Malaysian society into the international capitalist economy and global cultural reforms.

The key issues for women are associated with those reforms and risks that have emerged as a result of globalisation. These include rapid urbanisation and industrialisation which have been instrumental in increasing levels of environmental pollution and present serious threats to the health and well-being of the population in general and women in particular. An unstable economy also seriously undermines health and wellbeing leaving the country's poor to suffer the consequences of sudden depreciation of the currency.

Women in Malaysia face not only all the problems of women in developing countries such as Ghana and Malawi, but they also face the problems of a rapidly modernising world and so straddle the traditional and the modern which may not be a very comfortable place to be.

In the next chapter we travel to the ultimate in modernity – the United States of America. There we will explore the experiences of women who live in a society that has wealth, high technology, excellent transport systems and the most modern health care facilities in the world and yet find the reduction of maternal mortality a continuing challenge.

Chapter 6

Experiences of childbirth in America

During its history, the United States of America has been a country of extreme contrasts and abrupt changes. Most Americans face alternatives presented by such polarities as open immigration and 'jealous islands of tradition' (Erikson, 1977: 258); outgoing internationalism and defiant isolation; boisterous competition and self-effacing cooperation; and many others. For Erikson, the influence of the resulting contradictory metaphors on the development of individual identity probably depends on the coincidences of nuclear ego-states with critical changes in the family's geographic and economic chances.

American sociologist Robin Williams Jr (1970) summarised the values that he found were especially prominent in the USA. Among them were:

- Equal opportunity (Americans tend to feel that everyone should have equal opportunity to get ahead and are individually responsible for their own successes or failures).
- Achievement and success (Americans are oriented towards achievement and success, with one's degree of success typically measured by occupational achievement and level of material wellbeing).
- Activity and work (Americans are oriented towards work and like to keep active).
- Efficiency and practicality (Americans like quick, effective, and practical solutions to problems).
- Freedom (Americans strongly believe that individuals should have the right to free expression).

Bellah et al. (1985) agreed with Williams (1970) that Americans believed that success was determined by material wellbeing; that individuals should be free from having other people's values, ideas or lifestyles forced on them from arbitrary authority of others at work, in the family or in government; and that justice was largely a matter of equal opportunities. Ideally everyone should have the right to pursue whatever he or she understood as happiness as long as the rights and wellbeing of others were not harmed.

Bellah and his associates concluded that American culture emphasised individualism more than many other societies. Individualism in the American context is the belief that people had a right to think for themselves, to live their lives as they saw fit and to express themselves on the basis of their own opinions. This belief was strong in the USA and Bellah and his colleagues suggest that it lies at the very heart of American culture. The question is what this means for, and to what extent these values apply to, women in childbirth within American society.

American women's lives

The 1995 Census (US Bureau of Census, Department of Commerce Economics and Statistics, 1995), showed that the population of the United States was 134 million women and 128 million men. At the youngest ages (under 15 years), boys outnumbered girls by a ratio of 1.05:1. The male lead continued until 30 years old, when the situation reversed.

American women were racially and ethnically diverse. Of 134 million women, 83 per cent were white, 13 per cent were black, 4 per cent were Asian and Pacific Islanders, one per cent were American Indian, Eskimo and Aluet and 10 per cent were Hispanic (of any race).

American women experienced dramatic changes over the last four decades of the twentieth century. They increasingly delayed marriage and childbirth to attend college and establish careers. The median age at which women married for the first time was 24.5 (Bureau of Census). Between 1970 and 1994, the proportion of persons aged 30 to 34 years who had never married tripled from 6 to 20 per cent for women and from 9 to 30 per cent for men. For those aged 35 to 39, the corresponding increases were from 5 to 13 per cent and 7 to 10 per cent. These changes, according to the US Bureau of Census, (1995), have contributed to:

- More and more women living alone. Over this period, the number doubled from 7 to 14 million. For almost every age group, the percentage of women who lived alone also rose. The exception was the 65 to 74 age group, where the percentage remained statistically unchanged.
- More families being maintained by women without a husband. The proportion rose from 11 per cent of all families in 1970 to 18 per cent in 1994. They constituted 48 per cent of black families and 14 per cent of white families in the latter year.
- A large proportion of births were out-of-wedlock. About 26 per cent of babies born in 1994 were born out-of-wedlock. Of black women who gave birth in 1994, 66 per cent were unmarried, compared to 19 per cent of white women and 28 per cent of Hispanic women.

College enrolment of women was nearly that of men, although they still chose subjects of study that were different from those of men and less likely to lead to higher paid jobs (US Department of Commerce Economics and Statistics, 1995; US Department of Labor, 2001). While there are increasing numbers of women going into engineering, for example, fields such as health, particularly nursing, education, psychology, fine arts and foreign languages continue to be the major choices for women despite the increase in the fields that offer higher financial remuneration.

America is a country that epitomises the modern ideal. Modernity, indeed, some would argue postmodernity, and consumption appear to be a major part of American identity. Throughout the contemporary world there is a general recognition that the world we live in is dominated by capitalism. The degree to which this is diluted by alternative ideas such as socialism has diminished significantly since the late 1970s. While this may be true, Miller (1997: 2) argued that there has been a fundamental and significant change in the concept and practice of capitalism with the increasing centrality of consumption rather than production. We have moved away from a time when manufacturers made the goods first and then sought the markets to a time when retailers, the public and the media tell manufacturers what to produce. In many ways this is the current experience in childbirth with the advent of market forces in hospitals and among medical practitioners. In America this is exemplified in some ways by the development of home-like birth centres. In another way, what we are seeing now is that childbirth itself has become a commodity. Acts of consumption represent ways of fulfilling desires that are identified with highly valued lifestyles. Consumption is the material realisation, or attempted realisation, of the image of the good life and yet women are constantly depicted as being passive recipients of the market forces and prey not only to the power of the advertising genius of multinational companies but to the power of the obstetric industry.

Consumers, according to Miller (1997: 4), turn out to be among the most active players in the construction of the commodity from its inception. They are constantly involved through their reactions to branding (for the purposes of this argument, the branding referred to here is that of technological birth), and to advertising and strategies of selling, especially from obstetricians. There are times, however, when consumers are, in a sense, absent at key stages when one might expect them to occupy centre stage. For example, in advertising and marketing technological or no-technology birth the intense atmosphere of competition sometimes creates a fixation on rival ideals and organisations that pushes out any interest in or concern for the consumer. Obstetrics constantly justifies what it does in the name of the consumer, and in the belief that it understands the behaviour of the consumer. Similarly, consumers constantly credit obstetrics with the power of determining what they do as consumers.

Freidman (1989) argued that consumption is an aspect of broader cultural strategies of self-definition and self-maintenance. In these terms 'cultural' is equivalent to 'specificity' as in a specific structure of desire expressed in a specific strategy of consumption that defines the contours of a specific identify. Strategies of consumption, however, can only be truly grasped when we understand the specific way in which desire is constituted. And we shall assume for the time being that the latter is a dynamic aspect of the formation of personhood. This argument is in line with the four cultural types (hierarchist, egalitarian, isolationist and individualist), identified by Douglas and Thompson and discussed in chapter 2. Women's values and beliefs influence what they consume and consumption plays a significant part in defining social groups and individuals. The act of identification, the engagement of the person in a higher project, is in one sense an act of pure existential authenticity, but, to the degree that it implies a consumption of self-defining symbols that are not self-produced but obtained in the marketplace, the authenticity is undermined by objectification and potential decontextualisation. Distinction between individuals and groups is not merely for show but is a genuine vehicle which always comes from outside, a source of wellbeing and fertility and a sign of power. Members of the group can identify everyone's social or professional rank in a crowd by their outward appearance. Thus engagement authenticates, its consumption de-authenticates. The only authentic act inside such a system is an act that encompasses both the authentic and its commodification, that is, an engaged cynicism, a distancing that is simultaneously at one with the world. The following story exemplifies the struggle for authenticity through lifestyle choice.

The egalitarian struggle for authenticity

Grace's story

I am not a midwife – well not in the sense that I deliver babies. If the definition of the word 'midwife' is 'with woman' – then I am a midwife since I work with women. I do not have a midwifery qualification though, in the sense that I went to school and took exams. No – no-one would recognise me officially as a midwife I suppose.

At present I am a family nurse practitioner and I run a number of different programmes for pregnant women. Some of these have drug- and alcohol-related problems, using crack and cocaine, as well as those using heroin. Some have HIV/AIDS or other sexually transmitted disease. Others suffer with abusive relationships and many others are trying to raise children on their own. I see a high number of teenage pregnancies and quite a number of rape and incest victims in my clinic. A number of women have criminal records for different offences – prostitution, drug-related theft, etc. We are also seeing ever-increasing numbers of homeless women.

I see part of my role as an advocate for women's health issues and as working toward a comprehensive health policy for women and children – of all races – in this country. The problems change and grow. Poverty gets worse. We simply do not have an adequate health policy in the US. I believe the political atmosphere is hostile to women and children and a lot of my energy goes into advocating for the community and teaching. I talk to groups about what is going on in terms of public health; where the money is and how it is used or not. I let people know about the latest bills that might affect them. I talk to my community about how we need to become more politically motivated. We need to be present and vocal at public meetings because if we don't women and babies will continue to die or be damaged. Just as many women die now as before abortion was legalised. We cannot be silent in the face of such issues. I campaign to change whatever needs changing – take pollution for example. The sanitation hereabouts is not ideal – much of the city in which black people live is little more than a shanty town. Contaminated water supplies from raw sewage is not uncommon. This puts children and women at risk. The city is not sufficiently interested to repair worn out and broken drains and pipes and the people cannot afford to. Something has to be done.

Another area where I am concerned to make a change is in relation to technology in childbirth. We were told that technology would reduce mortality rates, but it didn't, and it made the rate of maternal morbidity rise in my view. I talk about this trend to women in my community. I let them know what the medical establishment is promoting and why. I believe that they are seeking to control the uterus and its contents and by so doing ultimately gain control over the woman. That's what I think and I will work towards better health and childbirth policies for women, especially for women of colour.

(Grace, Pennsylvania, 1995)

Erikson (1977) believed that whatever one may consider a truly American trait could be shown to have its equally opposite characteristic, although this is also probably true for all 'national identities'. The process of American identity formation appeared to support individual identity development provided that person preserved an element of deliberate tentativeness of autonomous choice. Thus functioning Americans, as heirs to extreme contrasts and abrupt changes, base their final identity on some tentative combination of dynamic polarities such as migratory and sedentary, individualistic and standardised, competitive and cooperative, piety and freethinking, rigidity and vacillation, responsibility and cynicism, and so on.

While extreme elaboration of one or the other of these poles can be seen in regional, occupational, and character types, Erikson's (ibid.) analysis revealed that this extremeness contained an inner defiance against implied, deeply feared, or secretly hoped for, opposite extremes.

Consequently, to leave choices open, Americans, on the whole, live with two sets of 'truths'. A set of religiously pronounced political principles of a highly puritan quality, and a set of shifting metaphors which indicate what, at a given time, one may get away with on the basis of little more than a hunch, a mood, or a idea. Thus, the same person may have been exposed in succession or alternatively to sudden decisions expressing the metaphors for example, 'Let's get the baby out of there' and again, 'Let's give the woman a chance'. Both of these conform to different myths of childbearing. The former would be an example of the myth that women's bodies are unpredictable and that birth must be controlled. The latter referring to the myth that labour and childbirth are normal events in women's lifecycles and that their bodies are robust.

Birth metaphors can be sufficiently convincing to those involved to justify their actions whether within or outside the law regardless of any pretence at logic or principle. These metaphors pervade public opinion in courts, in corner stores, and through television, films and the daily newspapers. In principles and ideas too, a polarity seems to exist on the one hand between intellectual and political elite which, always mindful of precedents, shield a measure of coherent thought and indestructible spirit, and, on the other hand, a powerful 'mobocracy' which seems to prefer changing metaphors to self-perpetuating principles. This was borne out during my fieldwork and data collection. Individuals and organisations appeared to swing between taking risks and avoiding risks, as expressed in the desire to try new things whilst fearing the consequences of failure. For practitioners in medicine and professional midwifery under the control of bureaucratic systems, however, erring toward conservatism and defensive practice was their only option. Individuals may hold polarised views but systems, especially hierarchical and bureaucratic systems, tend to err on the side of conservatism. System administrators tend to avoid setting precedents in the light of increasing pressure from the public, law courts and the media, as well as the scrutiny of the monitoring systems. In this context creativity and risk taking diminishes. The following story illustrates this point.

Camellia's story

Camellia is a home birth midwife and breast-feeding counsellor working in Texas.

The labour/delivery/recovery room set-up in the hospitals in my area is now the standard birth facility in Houston except for large charity hospitals. Women are told they can use the jacuzzi, shower, ambulate, eat, drink, etc. As a breast-feeding counsellor and midwife (home birth) I will tell you that I have met many women who feel disillusioned in that they could not use those facilities because their water broke, they were too far along, they were not far enough along, in labour, etc. I have gone to hospital-based 'Lamaze' (doctor obedience classes) and was even told that women with epidurals can walk and use the jacuzzi and not have an IV or shave or episiotomy, etc. The 'Lamaze' classes provided by the hospitals have merely become a tool of the hospital to indoctrinate couples into hospital routines! As for the women I have never met any woman who has been able to meet the hospital's criteria for any of the extras other than maybe a 'free' car seat for the baby.

(Camellia, Texas, 1995)

Fast birth: time as the dominant paradigm

For many American nurse-midwives, doctors and women, women's bodies are viewed as unpredictable within the context of the dominant 'body as machine' ideology that leads to a belief that childbirth is only normal in retrospect; therefore most women experience childbirth as a process that is fundamentally risky. This, in turn, leads to a high degree of instrumentalism in childbirth. The power of the middle-class, hierarchical, American child-birth hegemony is such that these notions are being transmitted globally and have an impact upon how women experience birth in countries which have been penetrated by Western knowledge, practices and technology. A some-what cynical view might be that like most technicians, doctors themselves are subject to productivity imperatives. Like servicing a car, each mechanic is paid for the total 'job'. The more technology involved in the job, the greater the fees that can be charged. More experience leads to expertise and a reputa-tion in undertaking technically complicated jobs attracts a greater number of clients.

The medical fraternity, according to Davis-Floyd, (1992: 46) as a con-sequence of their own initiatory rights of passage, are significant inculcators and 'enforcers' of the dominant belief system established on the generally accepted and approved American biomedical 'cures' that are based on sci-ence, effected by technology, and carried out in institutions founded on prin-ciples of patriarchy and the supremacy of the institution over the individual.

The shape of the social world affects ways of thinking about that world. This shape also includes concepts of time. In turn, people's conceptions become part of that social world insofar as they act towards things in terms of how they think about them. This is the connection between social percep-tions and the way people actually behave. This can be illustrated in the thinking and behaviour towards women's social roles, especially in regard to childbirth. This dominant view, however, may not be universal. A number of alternative groups adhere to different ideological and religious views of the world. The Amish society is an example of such an alternative approach, discussed later in this chapter.

Birth territory: where women birth

1. Birthing in the hierarchical model

In the latter-day context developing on from the mechanical model, Glennon (1979: 23) saw American society as essentially a technocratic society. Technocracy implies a social order in which all things are accommodated to the needs of science and technology – and their by-product, bureaucracy. Such a society finds itself more and more bureaucratised and run according to the dictates of scientism. In a technocratic society a cult of experts gains influential advocates, and ever-larger areas of life are drawn into its scope. Child rearing, lovemaking, sexuality, face and body language, ways of arguing and similar 'human' concerns are handed over to the experts for diagnosis and prescription.

People are subject to their social environment and America is a country that functions at high speed. It is the fast world described by Freidman (1999: 7). My observation of life in America was that people functioned at top speed and expected all things to be undertaken quickly, for example, fast food, instant banking, shopping channel and next day delivery, electronic mail rather than postal mail. It is a country that seems to resist delays in gratification and doctors and women in childbirth exist within the context of this fast world, as they do in the United Kingdom. The clock dominates our every action. Thus the ritual processes traditionally concerned with childbirth have been squeezed out by those generated by the dominance of time, for example, induction of labour, augmentation of labour, 'partograms' on which vaginal examinations are recorded to plot the progress of the labour, episiotomies, instrumental deliveries and caesarean section.

Childbirth in America, like many other human accomplishments, is in many ways a product of its technology. The artefacts of parturition, the utilitarian and ritual objects, instruments, and equipment necessary for a culturally proper management of labour and delivery constitute a significant part of America's birthing system. Methodologically, artefacts possess a quality that recommends them as vehicles for gaining access to a specific way of doing birth: in contrast to such intangibles as conceptualisations or expectations or attitudes, artefacts are visible and can be manipulated and are thus directly available for the practitioner's utilisation and the investigator's observations, for the asking of questions about them, for listening to talk regarding them, and sometimes, even, for gaining firsthand experience in using them. The collection of physical objects considered here includes not only 'obstetric tools' but all items recognised by participants as appropriate to doing birth. Thus, a talisman to ward off evil spirits is as important an object as the birthing stool or the presence of a delivery attendant is as important as the utensil with which the umbilical cord is cut.

Birthing systems overwhelmingly prescribe an appropriate place for giving birth. Jordan (1993: 67) considered that there were generally two kinds of environments: birth location may be relatively specialised, or within the woman's normal sphere. In either case, the choice of location has significant consequences in the resources it makes available and in the kinds of social interaction it produces.

The practice of moving the woman to a delivery room during labour and transferring her to a special delivery table is no longer followed in the majority of hospitals in England. While for many professional practitioners, this may seem a trivial concession to hospital efficiency, it may in fact, have far-reaching consequences. Jordan (ibid.: 68) observed in practice and in reports of women, the often rushed and hectic transfer to a trolley, the dramatic wheeling down the corridor with intravenous tubes dangling, and the always awkward and often painful transfer from the trolley to the delivery table, often transforms a marginally tolerable situation into a scene of frightful panic, as is often portrayed in films and fictional television programmes. Because of the woman's intense concentration and often desperate attempts to maintain control over her contractions at this time, the extent of distress created by these transfers is not visible to medical personnel. Jordan was impressed by the consistently angry remarks volunteered by women weeks later when they viewed their transfer to the delivery table on her video. To quote one of Jordan's research subjects:

> That was the most terrible part of the whole thing. I couldn't say any-thing because I was afraid I'd fall apart and I knew I had to get on that table to have that baby. But Jesus, why did they have to do that to me?
>
> (quoted in Jordan, 1993: 68)

From my own discussion with women who had had childbirth experiences in high technology settings, they often reported some years later an intense anger over being made to move at such a critical point in their labour.

Clare's story

Clare recalls the birth of her baby some five years after the event.

It was as if I was on a conveyer belt being moved along the assembly line in a factory. I had completed one section or rather one section had been completed, it had little to do with me as a person, it was the nurse's success – not mine – that I had reached this point. I could then be moved on to the next operator – the doctor – for the next part of the production process. It was humiliating and embarrassing. The white hospital gown open for all to see the big socks they made me wear. It was so undignified. Shifting from the trolley to the narrow delivery bed. I didn't think I would fit. Also the gap between the trolley and the bed seemed to be huge – I thought I would fall between them. It was terrifying. How could they expect me to be able to move about from one bed to another when I was trying to have a baby? It was awful.

(Clare, Pennsylvania, 1995)

Movement from the accustomed environment may have significant negative impacts upon women's physiological and behavioural responses. Besides transfer to a different location, crowding, fear, excessive noise, and newborn separation have been shown to produce negative reactions in women (see Odent, 1984).

American obstetric wards have traditionally been designed with a view to organisational efficiency and central availability of the resources of medical technology. From women's point of view, obstetric wards of most large American hospitals have a universally clinical atmosphere, the kind of environment that, if it is familiar at all, is familiar as a place of illness and suffering, a place for patients. Furthermore, the only appropriate place for the labouring woman is the patient's place – the bed. It is noteworthy that stand-ard hospital procedure gets the woman to her bed as quickly as possible and works to assure that she stays there.

Typically, following admission, an intravenous infusion is started and often an electronic fetal monitor attached. Either one of these procedures results in immobilising the woman on her hospital bed. Walking around during labour, encouraged as physiologically and psychologically beneficial in Europe, is considered unsafe in America. Although the rhetoric of mobility in labour has been incorporated into most American hospitals, it is often rendered physically difficult, if not impossible by the intravenous fluid tubes and moni-tor leads. Consequently, women are not only confined to the labour room and hospital bed, they are prevented from seeing what is happening around them to make sense of the noises they hear. People walking by in the hallway, trolleys being pushed, the clanging of instruments, strange faces coming into their field of vision from time to time, voices, screams, baby cries – against the background of their own increasing discomfort, all these contribute to a sense of disorientation, anxiety, and fear of what is to come. The women I encountered, however, held a medical view that the proper conduct of birth might be expected to be in the hospital setting because it would provide a sense of security, reassurance and trust for the childbearing woman, her partner and family. It is a trust that is sometimes betrayed.

According to Clare (research participant, 1995), most obstetric wards were designed without facilities for non-patients. Thus, there was, not only con-ceptually but also physically, no place for non-specialist participants who might act as the woman's companion, although the situation has been modi-fied in recent years in many American hospitals. It has become increasingly common for the labouring woman to be accompanied by the baby's father, a relative or a friend (Clare, Nurse-Midwives Focus Group, October 1995).

Most power-defining encounters take place on the doctor's territory where they can control the local resources and the power to use them at their discretion (Mary, Nurse-Midwives Focus Group, October 1995). Apart from this more obvious influence of territory control, there were more subtle interactional consequences, such as issues, for example, as who is guest and who is host, that influence participants' perceptions of what they are able to do, and thereby affect the tone of the interactions.

In the 1990s, when so many American women were educated for childbirth and gave birth consciously, with little pain (as a result of the extremely common use (80 per cent) of epidural anaesthesia (Mary, Nurse-Midwives Focus Group, October 1995), physicians increased their accountability to the awake and aware woman for undertaking proper procedures, giving explanations, and justifying their actions. But the language of the explanation like the territory in which they gave it, was still theirs to manipulate and the woman's to struggle to understand.

One of the most significant consequences of any system's choice of birth location is that this choice assigns responsibility for the course of labour and credit for its outcome. In American hospital deliveries, responsibility and credit were clearly the physician's. This became visible in the handshakes and 'Thank you' and 'Good work' compliments to the doctor by someone qualified to judge, that is another doctor, or perhaps the nurse. Typically, nobody thanks the woman. In the common view, she had been delivered, (passive role) rather than given birth (active role). In the home setting, by contrast, the initiative remains in many ways with the woman and her family. The birth is their choice, their problem, their task and will finally be their achievement.

The emperor's new clothes – re-dressing the hierarchical model of childbirth

The birth-centre phenomenon was a concept that was developed in response to a demand from educated, well-informed women who began to reject the routine application of technology and the depersonalised care provided in hospitals during labour and birth. They looked for doctors or midwives to attend them at home where they would feel free to move about, take nourishment and be within the closeness of their family while they laboured and gave birth. At that time (in the 1970s) there were almost no professionals willing to attend births at home in most parts of the United States.

Following closely on the heels of the birth centre development came the in-hospital alternative birth centre in direct competition. One can only assume that considerable funds were directed towards attracting women back into hospitals to give birth. In regard to the territory issue, hospital birthing rooms were not much more of an improvement over the labour and delivery room. The woman still gave birth in an unfamiliar environment attended by unfamiliar people, a guest on someone else's territory with few rights and fewer resources. While more flexibility was allowed in such things as position in labour, real decision-making power remained with medical personnel. In important ways, the woman still did not own the birth. One could characterise the introduction of birthing stools as a token de-medicalisation and a fairly superficial response to public demands for change. What was important, however, was that women responded very favourably to birthing rooms. They described the security they derived from the nearness of medical resources as an important factor in their positive experiences. We see, then, that for these women the most salient evaluation criterion remained the medical definition of what constituted safety, which alerts us to the fact that the definition of birth remained fundamentally unchanged.

Linda's story

Linda is a nurse in an in-hospital birth centre.

The topic of hospitals renaming regular labor and delivery areas birth centers, dressing them up with nicer furniture, etc., and thus misleading the public (and statistics gatherers) is a subject near and dear to me. I am a nurse in an in-hospital birth center which was created almost 10 years ago as a 'real' alternative to the existing labour and delivery ward (L & D). Without going into a lot of detail, I thought you might be interested in the fact that within the past two years our hospital has updated the L&D (definitely needed!), and advertised themselves as a Birthing Center (rather similarly named to our unit – The Birth Place) and thus they compete now with themselves!!! Worse yet, many of the care providers who have delivered with us very happily for 9 years are telling parents that there really isn't any difference because in both places you deliver in the same room, and can have early discharge if you want. Somehow they miss the major difference in philosophy – we treat birth as a normal, physiologic activity with the family paramount; it is still seen as a patient-related medical activity in the hospital, even in low risk situations.

(Linda, USA, 1995)

As in Lisa's birth, following, the thin veneer overlaying environmental change masquerades as profound change in childbirth philosophy and practice, and hides the artefacts of conventional American birth traditions. From the perspective of childbirth ecology birth location must be treated as an integral part of birthing systems. Apart from displaying to various degrees the attitudes to childbirth, the nature and layout of the birthing room tends to shape interactions between the participants and, consequently, the support available. Underlying these interactions and experiential consequences, we find that assignment of responsibility and credit for birth remain with the dominant medical fraternity. Technocracy legitimates the notion that science should serve productivity and bureaucratic administration by concentrating on the prediction and control of human behaviour. It provides sophisticated rationales to mask the use of humans as 'objects' in research or for example, childbirth (Glennon, 1979: 23). These rationales, however, accept a view of human behaviour that is intrinsic to a technocratic world-view – that all human processes can be explained, predicted and controlled by scientific investigation and technological manipulation. Moreover, technocracy implies the pervasive influence of instrumental orientations. Private and public spheres alike are approached technologically. Childbirth and child rearing, among other things of the same ilk, reflect the acceptance of instrumental assumptions in everyday life. The following rather extended account has been included to illustrate a number of issues: first the pervasive instrumentalism underlying the attempt to provide a home-like experience; second, to show how thin the veneer of the home-like environment is, and third to demonstrate the pressure upon the nurse-midwife to regress to the dominant conservative model of birth, regardless of her personal convictions.

Lisa's story

Lisa was a woman in her late thirties who had been admitted to the in-hospital birthing centre for a home-like birth. She graduated in 1985 from a College in New York with a degree in biology and pursued a career in medical research. She married at the age of twenty-five and had recently celebrated her 39th birthday. Here she is looking forward to the birth of her first child.

At the hospital Lisa entered the tastefully designer-decorated entrance hall with its pretty pictures of the countryside depicting the changing seasons. Three women in white dresses, white caps and white shoes, giving the impression of sterility and purity, were standing near the desk in the middle of the room chatting to each other.

The delivery suite looked even friendlier. Subtle terracotta walls and rust-coloured carpeting eliminated any preconceived ideas about sterile hospital surroundings. In the waiting room there was a fish tank and large plants to aid relaxation. There was even music playing. But that was where the home-like atmosphere ended.

Lisa and her husband were escorted into the delivery room. She sat on the delivery bed and was handed a gown to put on. Once changed, Lisa began to wander around the room, pausing only when she had a contraction. She returned to the delivery bed at the request of the nurse-midwife for an internal examination. Once on the bed the nurse-midwife took the opportunity to set up the external monitor to record the fetal heart and strength of the contractions.

There was the hollow pounding of a baby's heart – it sounded as if it were beating inside a metal tunnel. The fetal heart monitor stood next to the delivery bed. It was attached to the infant by way of red and green wires that disappeared into Lisa's vagina. Into her left wrist was flowing an infusion of a clear liquid as a substitute for energy foodstuff. Lisa lay absolutely still with her eyes closed. She had had some medication for pain and was drowsing between contractions.

The nurse-midwife turned first to the machine, and picking up the long strip of paper that poured out of it, examined the graphed recordings that ran its length. Absently she asked Lisa how she was doing, absently she acknowledged the small sign and a hesitant, 'Okay', and then, finally having satisfied herself with the recordings, she turned to look at Lisa. She adjusted the band around her abdomen. Like most monitoring tools, it inhibited Lisa's movements. Patting her arm, the nurse-midwife explained that the doctor would be along shortly. Meanwhile, Lisa's husband, James, was watching the basketball game on television.

Lisa suddenly tensed and all eyes turned to the monitor to watch the progress of the contraction. Even Lisa's eyes closely followed the increase and then decrease in the strength of the contraction. When it was over she sighed and closed her eyes again. No one looked at her. The nurse-midwife, doctor and Lisa's husband were too busy planning the next phase of the operation. A contraction suddenly exploded onto the screen. It looked like an expulsive contraction but she was not yet ready to push. The medical team decided that it was necessary to undertake an internal examination to assess the stage of labour. Upon completion they decided that Lisa could start pushing with her next contraction. As soon as the contraction began a few minutes later, Lisa's husband, nurse-midwife and doctor all began 'encouraging' her to push. Lisa screwed up her face and grunted. 'Push! Push! Take a deep breath, hold it, pushhhhhhhhhhhh-hhhhhhhhhhhhhh'. She clearly didn't feel the contraction or feel like pushing because of the regional anaesthetic she'd had earlier. They chanted at the top of their voices. The noise in the delivery suite was tremendous.

The doctor stepped towards the delivery bed and stared at the monitor. He didn't look at, or speak to, Lisa but greeted James cordially. 'Let's get her ready', he said pleasantly. The nurse-midwife began to reveal the hidden equipment around the room. As if by magic, the room transformed into a space-age technical laboratory. The doctor and nurse-midwife slipped on caps, gowns, goggles, masks and gloves.

Lisa was rolled awkwardly into the delivery position. Her legs were placed in leg stirrups and bound securely for safety reasons. The nurse-midwife spread a drape over each leg and then the doctor stepped forward to place the last drape over Lisa's body. The lamps in the room flashed on and the room made its final transformation into an operating theatre.

The doctor hadn't spoken to Lisa or touched her except to put the needle into her perineum. Now he picked up a pair of scissors and performed an episiotomy. Several contractions later, the baby's head emerged. The doctor slipped his fingers under the baby's chin to feel for the cord. With the next contraction, Lisa pushed and the baby's body was delivered. The baby was separated from his mother and taken away to the resuscitaire to be examined by the paediatrician. A heat lamp went on over the baby and a small plastic suction tube was passed down his throat. Without a word, the paediatrician handed the baby over to the nurse-midwife who trimmed his cord, wiped his face and weighed him. After a time, the newborn was handed to his mother for a few minutes before being put in a cot and taken to the nursery.

(an observed birth at Williamsport, Pennsylvania, 1995)

Ritual processes at work

There are several points at which ritual processes are enacted and myths of childbirth (see figure 6.1) are played out within Lisa's story. For the purpose of brevity, I will address only three ritual processes drawn from the work of Robbie Davis-Floyd (1992) and from personal observation and analysis.

The ritual purposes of electronic fetal monitoring (EFM)

Electronic fetal heart monitoring has become a 'normal' part of any hospital birth. Along with EFM came an increase in caesarean sections. The real reasons for increased caesarean-section rates amongst electronically monitored labours may well be obstetrician's impatience and nervousness. Studies have failed to demonstrate the benefits of routine EFM but doctors cite malpractice as a reason to persist. However since plaintiffs can and do portray the most trivial findings as ominous, the monitor recordings may be more harmful than helpful to the doctor. EFM appears to increase the risk of operative delivery without the justification of improved outcome. (Smith, Ruffin and Green, 1993: 1471–1481) Even in the high-risk case of prematurity, no benefits result from using electronic fetal monitors instead of periodic manual auscultation (Shy et al., 1990: 588–593).

So completely had the electronic fetal monitor 'mapped on' to Lisa's birth that both she and James began to feel that the machine itself was in control of her labour, indeed, even having the baby, while she was reduced to a mere onlooker.

In their response to the electronic fetal monitor, we can observe the successful conceptual synthesis between their perceptions of her birth experience and the technocratic model (Glennon, 1979).

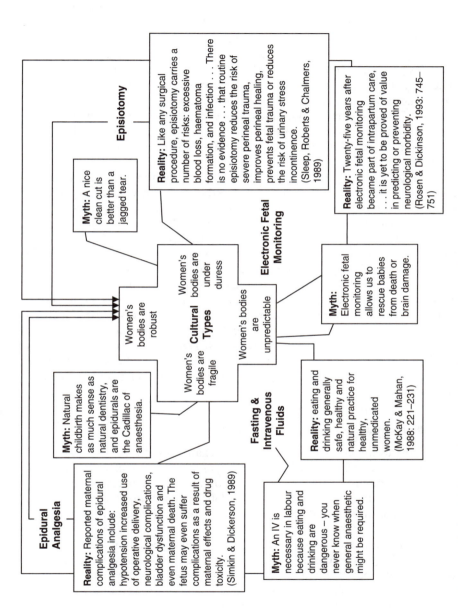

Figure 6.1 Myths of childbirth: obstetric myths and research realities in Lisa's story

According to Davis-Floyd (1992: 108) 'a common feature of rites of passage across cultures is the ritual adornment of the initiates with the visible physical trappings of their transformation'. In traditional societies the most deeply held values and beliefs of the society, are represented by such adornments as 'relics of deities, heroes, or ancestors . . . sacred drums or other musical instruments' (Turner 1979: 239). For Davis-Floyd, this perspective provides an insight into the symbolic significance of the 'EFM', a machine that has itself become a symbol of high-technology hospital birth. The electronic monitor, once attached, becomes the focal point of the labour, as nurses, midwives, doctors, husbands, and even the labouring woman herself become both visually and conceptually fixed on the machine, which in turn shapes their perceptions and interpretations of the birth process, as in Lisa's story.

The information produced by the electronic monitor is considered more authoritative than the information produced by the people involved generally and certainly more authoritative than women's knowledge, in particular. Jordan and Irwin (1989: 13 cited in Davis-Floyd, 1992: 108) define 'authoritative knowledge' as 'legitimate, consequential, official, worthy of discussion, and useful for justifying actions by people engaged in accomplishing a certain task or objective'. In early medical practice, doctors were completely dependent on their patient's description of their condition and on their own senses of touch and observation for knowledge about a complaint. With the invention of medical tests and procedures, medical practitioners became increasingly removed from the need to physically interact with their patients. The shift from a focus on the labouring woman herself to a focus on diagnosis by machine parallels the same movement in medicine, and reflects and perpetuates the cultural valuation of objective knowledge over subjective experience (Davis-Floyd, 1992: 108).

The ritual purposes of the vaginal examination

Within the technocratic model the vaginal examination is an important procedure that is carried out at regular intervals since the woman is only allocated a set amount of time in which to complete her delivery as defined by standard hospital policy. If the woman's labour is not progressing according to the standard tool of progress measurement, interventions must be instituted.

Cervical examinations are often quite painful especially when performed during the height of a contraction, as is often the case because more information can thus be obtained. The attending nurse or obstetrician normally performs these examinations. In teaching hospitals, however, any doctor in need of practice is likely to perform an examination sometimes without introduction or seeking permission.

For Davis-Floyd (1992: 112) any strategies the woman may have developed for coping with her labour in her own way will be disrupted by the frequent performance of vaginal examinations. Such examinations act as quality control mechanisms and are thus a necessary part of the industrial model of birth that attempts to reduce production time. These frequent production control checks are necessitated by the standardisation of modern birth, not by the physiological needs of the birthing woman and her child. In no other culture have such invasive, disruptive, and painful procedures been performed with such frequency and regularity as in the American hospital (Davis-Floyd, 1992: 112), although in Britain this practice has now also become routine. These frequent cervical examinations act to convince the labouring woman about the significance of time, about the suspected defectiveness of her own body, and about her lack of status and power relative to the hospital staff (the institution's representatives) and the institution (society's representative).

Painful cervical examinations also function as part of the ritual process in creating impersonal hazing of the initiate to ensure the complete breakdown of her category system so that she will be as psychologically open to the reception of the messages imparted by her birth experience as possible. These examinations powerfully intensify the process of symbolic inversion begun earlier. Imagine the messages conveyed to the woman by a series of strangers invading her body. For as Davis-Floyd states, this must approach the extreme opposition of a woman's usual ideas of an appropriate relationship between herself and society, an extreme that will ultimately be reached on the delivery table with the lithotomy position.

The ritual purposes of the lithotomy position

Many hospitals and obstetricians still insist on placing the woman about to deliver her baby in the lithotomy position. The woman lies with her legs in stirrups and her buttocks close to the lower edge of the table. She is thus in an ideal position for the attendant to deal with any complications which may arise (Oxorn and Foote, 1975: 110 cited in Davis-Floyd, 1992: 121). This position, in other words, is the easiest for performing obstetric interventions, including maintaining sterility, monitoring fetal heart rate, administering anaesthetics, and performing and repairing episiotomies (McKay and Mahan, 1984: 111). From this position the baby is born heading upwards towards the obstetrician. The supine position, however, is possibly the worst conceivable position for labour and delivery for both the woman and baby (see Balaskas and Balaskas 1983: 8; Humphrey *et al.*, 1973, 1974; Kurz *et al.*, 1982; McKay and Mahan 1984).

For Davis-Floyd (1992: 123) the lithotomy position completes the process of symbolic inversion that was set in motion when the woman was first put into the hospital gown on admission. Her normal bodily patterns of relating to the world have now been quite literally up-ended: her buttocks on the edge of the delivery table, her legs widespread, and her vagina completely exposed. 'As the ultimate symbolic inversion, it is ritually appropriate that this position is reserved for the peak transformational moments of this initiation experience: the birth itself' (Davis-Floyd, 1992: 123). The official representative of society, its institutions, and its core values of science, technology and patriarchy stand not at the woman's head nor at her side, but at her bottom, where the baby's head is beginning to emerge.

This, for Davis-Floyd, represents a total inversion, appropriate from a societal perspective, as the technocratic model promises that women can give birth with their cultural heads instead of their natural 'bottoms'. The cultural value is placed on the baby, who is emerging at the 'top' toward the obstetrician and indeed emerging upwards against gravity – struggling against and symbolically conquering nature. Conceptually speaking, the downfall of the initiate's category system is now complete. The lithotomy position expresses and reinforces the woman's now total openness to the new messages. One of those messages speaks so eloquently to her of her powerlessness and of the power of society at the supreme moment of her own individual transformation.

Obstetric practices and hospital childbirth policies deconstruct birth, then invert and reconstruct it as a technocratic process through hospital ritual procedures. Unlike most transformations effected by ritual, however, birth is not dependent upon the performance of ritual to make it happen. The woman is transported into a naturally liminal space that carries its own affectivity, through the physiological process of labour itself. Obstetric procedures and hospital policies take advantage of that affectivity to transmit the core values of American society to birthing women. The birth process will not be deemed successful from society's perspective unless the woman is properly socialised during the experience, transformed as much by the rituals as by the physiology of birth. Despite the power of these covert symbolic messages, the technocratic model of birth is overtly predicated on science. Sometimes there may be a divergence between scientific fact and actual practice, as in the case of the lithotomy position. Davis-Floyd (1992: 124) would urge us to either abandon or change the routine everyday practices in light of most compelling evidence even if that challenges accepted standard procedures.

This transformative process is neither inherently negative or inherently positive since every society has a need to socialise its members into the social norms. Relying on surveillance and sanctions to make them conform would be impractical. It is more practical for societies to socialise their members internally, by making them want to conform to societal needs. Every culture has developed rituals to ensure just that. Women, however, are not automatons. Despite the power of obstetricians and the dominant medical model, there is a resurgence of interest in midwifery in the United States as a counter-balance to medical supremacy.

2. Challenging the hierarchical model: the egalitarian model

By contrast, the midwifery model in the United States, which is essentially egalitarian in approach (Gibson, 1999; Idarius, 1999; Schlenzka, 1999) aims to empower women by assisting them to actively engage with the challenges of pregnancy and birth. Traditionally, midwives view pregnancy and birth as healthy, normal, everyday events, albeit ones that require supervision and care. In the midwifery model, the childbearing woman has the central role and the midwife watches over her, serves her, provides information and support, ultimately facilitating the birth process itself. Decision-making is collaborative and any intervention needed often begins with what the woman can do for herself. Often women in America study midwifery in hopes of becoming closer to other women; not just as friends, but with the goal of establishing support systems and creating community. The evolutionary social aspect of midwifery is that it motivates women to extend the responsibility they take in birthing to one another, breaking out of isolated nuclear families into networks of interdependent mothers and children, identifying and sharing their resources. Thus midwifery can be linked to social innovations such as the provision of childcare facilities in the workplace, and generally a more tolerant attitude towards women who try to interface family life with their careers.

Certainly the midwife appears to be an advocate of choice. Midwives in America vigorously defend the right of parents to choose their place of birth, as they fight for their own right to practise in a variety of settings. Hospital privileges are often denied midwives in the US and home birth is still controversial, although statistics have repeatedly shown home delivery to be as safe or safer than hospital birth (Duran, 1992; Mehl, 1977; Sullivan and Beeman, 1983).

Mary's story

Mary is a midwife practising in Pennsylvania.

My home delivery statistics were striking. I rarely did episiotomies. At first, I thought it might be accidental – that I'd had a run of women with favourable birthing bodies. In those first months of doing home deliveries, Lette and I watched women, 8 centimetres dilated, making coffee for us while cooking a family meal, bending and cleaning, making the bed, and stepping into the bathroom for a quick shower. We were used to American women in hospitals, 8 centimetres dilated, who believed they needed help to sip water.

(Mary, Pennsylvania, 1995)

The majority of women wanting midwifery care choose to give birth at home. Typical reasons include greater comfort and less intervention. Despite the resurgence of midwifery, midwives themselves are constantly under duress from the dominant medical system as the following extract illustrates.

Petra's story

Petra primarily worked in settings that served high-risk, low-income, multi-ethnic, multi-lingual women.

The actual work done with these women seemed to counter the contamination and warped values that the prevailing systems often reflected. I have worked in University settings, small county hospitals, large county hospitals, private medical units practices, and one midwifery practice. All used the hospital as the birthing setting. All situations competed with physician's caseloads.

Frequently I have had faculty appointments at large universities and have taught residents, medical students, midwifery students, nursing students, etc. The teaching role as a midwife is a balancing act between the client-midwife relationship and the learner's needs. At times I justified teaching as a process of 'humanizing' birth in the larger picture. Lately, it is a sense that I have to do it or lose my job, despite the fact that the physicians I am teaching are the ones who will go into practice and decrease my numbers, causing my layoff. Competition is healthy if the playing field is level. It is not for midwives, and more recently, specialists.

I went into midwifery twenty years ago. It was a passion to care for women and families in the birth process. I wanted my work to be integrated into my life. I wanted a community where I could be part of the web. Watch the babies grow. Nurture my own homestead. Raise my own family. Participate in community events. A slow and thoughtful life, I hoped.

It seemed there was a crossroads when I chose the route into midwifery those many years ago. I opted to be a Certified Nurse Midwife (CNM) because I didn't want to work underground which was the tone at that time. I hoped to be part of the process of change which would allow more women to be midwives in their home communities. I always supported the home as an appropriate birth setting. I do not relate to a nursing identity and never worked as a nurse. I helped set up birth centres in the seventies. I wanted a 'real' salary and benefits. It became increasingly clear that salary and benefits are a luxury if you want to practice out of the hospital or not to be on call the majority of your life. Now, midwifery seems polarized, when I felt we used to be sisters. I am at the end of my ability to compromise with the mainstream medical/midwifery scene.

(Petra, USA, 1995)

3. The isolate model of childbirth: the Amish society

In Lycoming County, I was privileged to meet with an Amish midwife, Mary, who invited me into her home and conveyed many birth stories from her years of practice as a lay midwife. Mary showed me a quilt that was embroidered by the mothers she had delivered. The first patch was made by the first delivery she conducted and had the name of the mother, father and child embroidered on it. Several generations later, Mary could point to the history of birth in that family, to all the siblings and relations that she had helped to birth over the years. It was a history not only of her life but that of the community she served. Such traditions are an important feature of the Amish community.

Mary belonged to the Old Order Amish who are among the most conservative descendants of the 16th-century Anabaptists. They are usually distinguished from the Amish Mennonites, Beachy Amish and the New Order Amish by their strict adherence to the use of horses on the farm and as a source of transportation, their refusal to allow electricity or telephones in their homes, and their more traditional standard of dress, including the use of hook-and-eye fasteners on some articles of clothing.

In the last century the Old Order Amish population grew very rapidly. In 1900 there were approximately 3,700 Amish in North America. By 1990 the estimated figure had increased to 127,800 (adult membership approximately 56,200). According to Erickson (1979) and her colleagues, the Amish were among the fastest-growing populations in the world at that time. They prohibit the use of contraception and have low infant mortality rates. The average Amish woman expects to have at least seven live births. Childbirth in Amish society is unheralded and taken as an everyday event as can be seen from the rather lengthy story that follows. The full text is provided here to act in juxtaposition to the story of Lisa's birth earlier in this chapter. The purpose of this will become clear in chapter 8 as I reflect on the case studies and attempt to draw some conclusions.

Ruth's birthing as told by Rachel

Rachel is an Amish midwife. She has worked in her community for more than thirty years.

Yesterday I delivered Ruth and Jacob's baby. Ruth had a bunch of things yet to do before she had her fifth baby, and she was especially determined to get into a quick bath. She had her husband running here and there, looking for various unspecified items. I think she was just keeping him occupied as usual. I asked her if she felt like pushing yet and she said no, she didn't, and besides she needed to have a bath. She'd been working in the field bundling up sheaves of corn right up until I arrived and her feet were dirty.

I'd set out my things in the bedroom, and sat down to read a magazine article about growing herbs. Ruth's husband, Jacob, brought in some things I needed, and just before he sat down, Ruth called from the bathtub, 'Ask Rachel if she wants any tea, Jacob'. I didn't, so he sat down to read the weekly newspaper that serves Old Order Amish communities. There wasn't a sound in the house except for the ticking of Ruth's clock.

She came out of the bathroom about ready to push. 'Come on, Jacob,' she said, 'let's go have this baby.'

Ruth and Jacob's bedroom was too warm, and Jacob opened a couple of windows just an inch or two. It began to rain outside the window, the wind gusted, the curtains billowed slightly at the window, and the smell of wet earth filled the bedroom. You can always count on deliveries on nights with thunder and lightning. We got Ruth settled on her bed, arranged her pillows, and her husband lit a bedside lamp. For a while, I massaged her feet and legs; her husband dusted his hands with talcum and rubbed his palms into the small of her back.

'Okay, Ruth. Let's get you up on your knees. We need to give those bones the best chance to spread for the baby's head.' Ruth sat with her bottom resting on her heels. 'That's good. I can see the baby's head now.' The baby came down the birth canal, turned, slid under the pubic bone, and then its head began to emerge. The perineum thinned. I put my fingers on the cap of the baby's head to keep it from coming too quickly, to give the perineum a chance to stretch. I asked Ruth to pant. The baby's head rotated and the perineum slipped over the brow of the face. 'There now, there, Ruth, there's your baby's head.'

Jacob came over to look over my shoulder. 'One more push for the body', I said. Ruth, not losing any momentum, surged one more time, and the baby was out. It started crying right away.

'It's a boy,' I said, putting the baby on the bed next to Ruth and covering him with a receiving blanket while I cleaned fluids from his nose and mouth. Ruth stayed on her knees, a small amount of blood pooling under her, then giving its standard warning with a narrow rush of fresh blood – the placenta followed. Ruth said little but drew the baby toward her, cuddling him at her side. Jacob said, 'This will make Grandma's forty-eighth grandchild – that is, if somebody hasn't beat us to it.'

Jacob cut the cord, we wrapped the baby a little better. I passed the baby to Jacob to carry about – 'leave his head a little lower than the rest of his body so that he won't choke on any mucus' – while I washed Ruth. She was shaking from having used up all her energy, so I covered her up with piles of family quilts and got her some apple juice.

Ruth and Jacob's baby would be called Caleb. I washed him, amusing Ruth with my conversation as I did, weighed him, and then put him back on the bed to check him. Telling him who he resembled, who the grandparents were, I dressed him and wrapped him in a blanket. I put him in the crook of his mother's arm and he started nursing.

I left Ruth and Jacob's house shortly after the baby started nursing at the breast. I said, 'Keep the baby warm and help him get gradually accustomed to the outside world. Let him sleep next to you. Don't worry, you won't roll over on him – you'll know he's there.'

(Rachel, Lycoming County, Pennsylvania, 1995)

In many communities the Amish have acculturated into the dominant culture to some extent. They have borrowed technology as well as ideas from their non-Amish neighbours. Examples of the former included the increase in the use of diesel or gasoline engines to provide power for machinery. Indoor plumbing, gas stoves, and refrigerators were found in more and more Amish homes. In some Amish homes secular as well as non-Amish religious print materials were found. Ideas which were not part of their culture are making their way into the Amish community. The following story exemplifies some of these changes.

Jennifer's story

Jennifer is a nurse-midwife working among the Amish.

I live in Indiana, which is a state where direct entry midwifery is a class D felony. I don't know anything about the statistics. Because we are illegal, it is very hard to get good statistics.

The Amish are regarded as quaint, picturesque, or with nostalgia, (the good old days), but they are mostly just women having babies, lots of babies. I had to learn practical things when working with the Amish. Lighting at night, no telephone if another client needs to talk to me, warming the house quickly, etc. The births, the babies, the sounds, the emotions, the beauty . . . it is all universal. 'My' Amish clients eat a lot of junk food, highly processed foods, and home grown foods full of pesticides. They wear polyester, use pampers, have a high percentage of hospital births, a high caesarean section rate, (also a very high hysterectomy rate) and don't breastfeed very long. Most of my work with them is trying to get them to have more prenatal care, better diets, to work less, especially postpartum (which is a losing battle), and to breastfeed longer, which besides being good for the baby, will help delay the return of menses, and consequently the next baby.

They are interested in that! I probably do one or two Amish births a month, three to five a month total, but not all of those are primary care. I work with two other midwives and attend births with them also, as much as I can.

(Jennifer, Indiana, 1995)

While acculturation is occurring, there was no evidence that Amish culture is on the verge of disappearing. In discussion during fieldwork, the Amish I encountered clearly understood the boundary between their culture and the non-Amish world. Where change was deemed to be necessary, as in the case of providing Mary with a telephone in her home, and, in some instances unavoidable, it was made cautiously and with a great deal of discussion.

Concluding comment

As has frequently been noted in respect of knowledge in technological cultures, the latent meanings implicit in bio-medicine lie in the very assertion that it is free from the influence of symbol and value. This is what a series of writers have referred to as the 'de-politicising' role of modern science (Barthes, 1973: 142ff; Habermas, 1971: 114; Marcuse,1972: 130) which is fundamentally conservative because it supports the status quo. While it is clearly naive to assert that medicine can be seen as the mere product of utilitarian social interest, its symbolic forms, like those of all human knowledge, express particular resolutions of more deep-seated paradoxes, and a world-view consonant with definite social interests.

I have attempted to demonstrate that childbirth in America is a process that emerges from a society that is based upon technocratic assumptions and a core value of individualism. Part of that process involves an increasing refinement of the use of technology in birth, but at the same time an expanded exposure of more women to instrumental childbirth in the drive to reduce mortality as an indicator of the country's wellbeing.

In this chapter I have argued that American midwives, doctors and women view women's bodies as unpredictable within the context of the dominant 'body as machine' ideology that leads to a belief that childbirth is only normal in retrospect; therefore most women experience childbirth as a process that is fundamentally risky; this leads to a high degree of instrumentalism in childbirth. The power of American hegemony is such that these notions are being transmitted globally and have impacted upon how women experience birth in countries penetrated by Western influence in terms of knowledge, practices and technology.

I acknowledge that these arguments are neither profound or novel. However they are significant, and an awareness of them can help midwives deal with some of the myriad complexities that are involved in childbirth both within their own culture and in others. To quote one of the respondents:

Sometimes a birth means so much more to a woman than anyone can know. It is not about having a cosy environment. If birth is examined deeply it can be seen that it is more than just a means to an end. A healthy mother and baby is, of course, the bottom line, but sometimes there are many other factors involved. In cases where anomalies not compatible with life are present some families will choose to birth at home. The risk is acknowledged but death and difficulty are emotional issues that touch the core of existence and sometimes those involved need to be in a place where they can deal with it in their own way. A hospital environment with its rules and routines often overlooks the inner needs that go beyond the nice wallpaper and rocking chair. The needs are for support, emotional and physical, for quiet and the chance to take their time. For a couple facing the inevitable death of their baby, being at home may mean having the chance to let their baby die in their arms as opposed to an isolate filled with wires and tubes. To be surrounded by people they know and trust. The kind of fast food prenatal care given to most women does not allow that kind of relationship to develop. While some improvement is being made in some areas of America, the dominant paradigm still prevails.

(Samantha, USA, 1999)

American society is a much more complex and geographically and culturally diverse country than I have described here. I was unable to explore all the different racial and cultural groups. Clearly issues of race, poverty and access to maternity care across the United States are important and have implications for childbirth and preparation of midwives. The research population in Pennsylvania, however, was largely Germanic in origin and relatively wealthy. The most significant contrast that I could draw was between the Amish and other women in Lycoming County that enabled me to examine childbirth and midwifery education from different standpoints. One interesting question I was unable to address was why it was that the Amish were protected so that they could pursue their religious and cultural practices including childbirth when the African-Americans were not. African-American lay midwives were outlawed and were unable to practise their traditional birthing practices.

Chapter 7

Experiences of childbirth in England

Contemporary British society is increasingly diverse and complex. Underlying this complexity are some basic structural elements, two of the most important of which are capitalist social relations and a culture of modernity in which social groups have very different social experiences. The major cause of the complexity of contemporary British society is, however, the speed of social change: Britain, like all modern societies, is a dynamic society. This dynamism originated from and is sustained by capitalist social relations. The pattern of ownership of the means of production, changes in the distribution of income and wealth, the increasing complexity and fragmentation of the class structure, and the growth of the welfare state are just a few of the factors that have radically altered British society. Indeed, capitalism by its very nature is an economic system that produces change and diversity, and a self-propelling, ever-accelerating kind of society.

Rapid economic change and cultural change are closely linked. While not necessarily welcoming it, many people positively seek change. This may not only occur at the individual level – moving to another town, changing job and buying new or different types of goods – but also occurs collectively, in the political sphere and in the neighbourhood. New social movements emerge from groups of people who collectively attempt to change the social world. Britain, in this sense, is an 'active' society. People believe and act as if they can alter the circumstances under which they live, to improve their own conditions and those of others.

Constant change and innovation generates a distinctive kind of social experience, which leads to uncertainty about the future, feelings of insecurity and anxiety, and a sense of bewilderment in negotiating everyday life. At the same time, such change brings about restlessness with permanence, seeking new experiences in pursuit of self-development, and a selfish concern with personal wellbeing. The contradictory modern experience generates particular personality types and threatens social instability as norms and behaviour change. Old values and practices are discarded as new kinds of fashions emerge, and traditional institutions are transformed.

Arguably, the modern experience has been amplified in the last three decades to the extent that the foundations of knowledge are subject to radical doubt; lifestyles become less uniform, social interactions less predictable, commitments less permanent and self-identities less fixed. Some sociologists refer to this as the postmodern condition (see for example, Lyotard, 1984; Harvey, 1989). Under the conditions of postmodernity people tend to be more experimental and less dogmatic, to adopt a playful attitude towards identities, images and meanings, to appreciate social and cultural variety, and perhaps to be increasingly tolerant of differences between groups.

While some of the possibilities for new experience and social experimentation associated with capitalist modernity are to be welcomed, others are not. The paradox is that we tend to acquire both the beneficial and the detrimental consequences simultaneously. For example, family relationships are changing, divorce is on the increase, there are increasing numbers of lone parents and growing social and economic insecurity. The growth of youth sub-cultures is equally typical of modernity. Unusual styles of dress, language, music and entertainment alter frequently as young people pursue distinctive, and new, group identities. Such styles are associated with a capitalist commercialism, which, in seeking to persuade people to buy more, encourages changes of fashion and allegiances to particular lifestyles.

In an important sense the experience of modernity is an urban phenomenon, an experience that is concentrated in cities where social relations are often described as being relatively impersonal, impermanent, varied and unpredictable. There are, however, urban centres where a sense of community survives with everyone knowing everybody else and where there are communally enforced rules of behaviour. This demonstrates the complexity of modern social experience. Complexity involves a multiplicity of experiences, and considerable diversity.

Diversity can also generate inequality and, possibly, conflict. The pursuit of equality, along with the pursuit of liberty, has been a fundamental pursuit to promote social change in Britain throughout the capitalist era. Social groups seeing themselves as unequally treated have organised together to improve their position.

The shape of the occupational structure has been changing in recent years, the numbers of manual workers declining, and the numbers of professional and semi-professional jobs increasing. This has come about as a result of industrial change, which inevitably affects class relations and the class structure. Moreover, according to Abercrombie *et al.* (2000) women have played a critically important part in the redefinition of the social division of labour since the late 1960s. There are more married women in paid work today than there have been at any time in the last century. The jobs that women have, however, tend to be relatively poorly paid and carry little authority. The segregation of men's work from women's work has its roots in the cultural stereotypes of women as in, for example, the unequal distribution of housework, in images of femininity which describe women as helpless and passive, and in male violence against women.

Similarly, the labour market intersects with cultural stereotypes to create a further social division, which is a source of social conflict between ethnic groups. Many members of ethnic groups, particularly those of Caribbean and Asian descent, even those born in Britain, experience social and material deprivation when compared with the Caucasian population. The presence in Britain of many different ethnic groups along with contemporary cultural products – family structure, food, music, religion – is symbolic of the diversity of culture and experience among different sections of the population. These differences are, however, frequently associated with inequalities, for example, black people tend to get poorer jobs and suffer the consequences of racism.

For Abercrombie *et al.*, the family is one institution, which exemplifies the degree of variety and complexity that characterises social experience in Britain, and one which illustrates the insecurity and instability of social relations in the contemporary world. A striking feature of the contemporary British family is the variety of forms it assumes. Besides distinctive household patterns of ethnic minorities that are often adapted from their particular religious and cultural traditions or the need to provide accommodation for newly arrived immigrant kinsfolk, there is a remarkable diversity of household forms among other sections of the population too. The dominant image of an 'average' family in contemporary Britain of a small, nuclear family of parents and dependent children is, in reality, becoming increasingly unusual. Changing attitudes to family and marriage have resulted in a rise in the numbers of single-person households, of one-parent families and of families formed by remarriage and step-parenting. Not only is the divorce rate high, but more couples are living together without getting married and are deciding to have children together while increasing numbers of people are opting to live by themselves. The overall fertility rates have declined, however, and this decline is most marked in women under 30 years as women choose to both delay childbirth and have fewer children (Office for National Statistics (ONS), 2000). The average age at which women in England and Wales gave birth during the study period was 29 years. The average age at birth of the first child was 27, although there are geographical variations. Women in the south were slightly older (average age 28 years) compared with an average age of 26 years for women in the north and Wales. The average age at second pregnancy was 30 years. In 2000, 52 per cent of conceptions were outside marriage compared with 42 per cent in 1989.

Teenage conception rates fell in the early 1990s but rose between 1995 and 1998. Between 1999 and 2000 the teenage conception rate fell by almost 1 per cent, from 62.9 to 62.2 conceptions per 1,000 women aged 15 to 19. The estimated number of conceptions to girls under 16, however, rose by 2 per cent from 7.9 thousand in 1999 to 8.1 thousand in 2000. About 70 per cent of those conceptions were to girls aged 15 years. The percentage of underage conceptions leading to an abortion increased from 53 in 1999 to 54 in 2000 (ONS, 2002). Teenagers are more likely to become pregnant if they live in poor urban areas. Inner city authority Southwark, for example, has five times the rate of conceptions amongst under 18s than the lowest rated authority, affluent Chiltern. According to statistics from the Office for National Statistics (ONS, 2000), girls are least likely to become pregnant in prosperous rural areas.

Britain is a highly urbanised society where the greater majority of women give birth in obstetric facilities, whether they are having normal or complicated births. The very nature of these facilities fosters a temptation to treat all births routinely with the same high levels of intervention as those required by women who experience complications. This can have a wide range of negative effects, some of them with serious consequences. These range from the sheer cost of time, training and equipment demanded by many of the methods used, to the fact that many women may be deterred from seeking the care they need because they are concerned about the high level of intervention. Moreover, women and their babies can be harmed by unnecessary practices. Staff in maternity units can be rendered dysfunctional if their capacity to care for women with complications is swamped by the sheer volume of normal births that present themselves. In their turn, those normal births are frequently managed with standardised procedures that can only be justified in the care of women with childbirth complications.

Childbirth in the United Kingdom is very similar to that in the United States of America with a few notable exceptions. The first is that midwives operate freely, under strict rules and codes of practice, but within the law in the UK. The second difference is that maternity services in the UK are concerned to provide women with choice, continuity and control in childbirth. These themes were to become a central force in the Changing Childbirth report (Department of Health, 1993). At least the rhetoric was one of choice, continuity and control – the reality was and is frequently very different. In many other respects childbirth in the UK is the same: technologically determined, scientifically driven and medically dominated. The experiences of women and midwives point out the seemingly paradoxical nature of discontent with maternity services in the UK given the continued fall in perinatal mortality. There are persistent calls from women, pressure groups and midwives for a balance between the safety considerations and the social aspects of childbirth. In the context of most health-care systems in the industrialised world, this is a radical perspective that recognises that childbirth is much more than a medical event.

Legally, women in the United Kingdom do not need to be under the care of an obstetrician during their pregnancy or childbirth. Instead they can opt for midwifery care or indeed, none at all.

Hierarchical and egalitarian: opposing approaches to childbirth

At first glance, childbirth in the UK has changed, but in two opposite directions. One is towards woman-centred, holistic care provided by midwives, and the other is towards increasingly high-technology obstetric management. Most childbirth in England takes place in hospitals. The increasing medicalisation of childbirth is one aspect of social change, and its effect is carried on throughout the continuum of women's lives. In an attempt to mediate across the divide midwives, women and obstetricians have more or less adopted a risk approach to childbirth. If a woman is deemed to be low risk then her care falls within the domain of the midwife and her choices are more extensive – her place of birth, labour carer, position and so on. If a woman is deemed to be high risk, then her care is more restricted and falls within the domain and control of the obstetrician. Risk assessment is based on probability – probability demands calculation. Because of the unpredictability of pregnancy and childbirth, the probability of something happening must, by default, be high – consequently all pregnancy and childbirth is risky.

Risk approach in childbirth: hierarchist model

Childbearing can be one of the most special events in a woman's life. It can also be one of the most dangerous (WHO, 1987). I would argue that this belief is too simplistic because if childbearing was dangerous of itself, then the human race would be extinct. The conditions under which women become pregnant and give birth play a significant part. Poverty is the leading culprit to complications of pregnancy and birth (Bergstrom, 1996).

The improvement in perinatal mortality rate in the United Kingdom that followed improvement in maternal health status unfortunately coincided with increasing obstetric management. It was then 'all too easy' to attribute the declining perinatal mortality rate to the benefits of obstetric management. The 'risk approach' to maternity care has dominated decisions about birth, its place, its type and the caregiver for decades (Enkin, 1995). The problem with many such systems is that they have resulted in a disproportionately high number of women being categorised as 'at risk', with a concomitant risk of receiving a high level of intervention in childbirth:

> Obstetricians ... have become convinced that the natural process of birth is fraught with dangers, which their increasingly sophisticated technological interventions are increasingly capable of minimizing. Amazingly, they have managed, without producing any valid supporting evidence, to persuade the majority of people, medical and lay, that they are right.
>
> (Tew, 1986: 659)

Relatively few people now believe that for healthy women, giving birth is a normal physiological process.

Obstetricians have used risk assessment to identify women who may have major medical difficulties during pregnancy or delivery. Typically, they label as 'high-risk' those women who become pregnant under 15 or over 40 years of age, who already have more than five children or a recent newborn, or who have health problems such as diabetes, heart disease, or hypertension. These assessments are used to encourage non-pregnant women in high-risk categories to practice effective contraception and to monitor pregnant women for special treatment and referral if necessary.

For Rooney (1992) the effectiveness of a risk-scoring system is measured by its ability to discriminate between women at high and low risk, that is by its sensitivity, specificity, positive and negative predictive value. Exact figures about the discriminatory performance of these risk-scoring systems, however, are difficult to obtain, although such estimations are made (Van Alten *et al.*, 1989; De Groot *et al.*, 1993). For example, defining obstetric risk by demographic factors such as parity and maternal height has a low specificity and therefore results in many uncomplicated deliveries being labelled as high risk. The specificity of complications in the obstetric history or in the present pregnancy may be much higher. The problem with this analysis however, is that consideration of other factors such as social, environmental and health factors are seldom included. Surveillance during birth cannot make up for a history of poor health, malnutrition and environmental hazards. Surveillance only leads to intervention after the fact and this is often of little value to the present pregnancy or birth. It is less than useful in terms of prevention. Antenatal surveillance cannot improve the present pregnancy or make up for poor health and malnutrition but WHO is suggesting that it is important to monitor women during labor and act on complications that arise at that time (WHO, 1999).

Obstetric risk assessment is a continuing procedure throughout pregnancy and labour because it is viewed that at any moment complications may become apparent and may induce the decision to refer the woman to a higher level of care. This is based on a view of childbirth in which the woman's body is unpredictable, under duress, and requiring structure (hierarchist approach). Within this categorisation, the midwife functions within the dominant medical domain and her roles are observing the conventions and maintaining the status quo of the medical paradigm (see figure 7.1). The language used is that of medicine. Women are seen as patients, birth is spoken of in terms of confinement, and women are expected to be passive. Medicine lays claim to authoritative knowledge and women's ways of knowing and knowledge of their bodies are regarded as inferior. Ultimately, women lose their identities and control as a result of the institutions' ritual processes, just as described in Lisa's story in chapter 6.

The prevalence of the concept of obstetric risk drives us towards a deficit

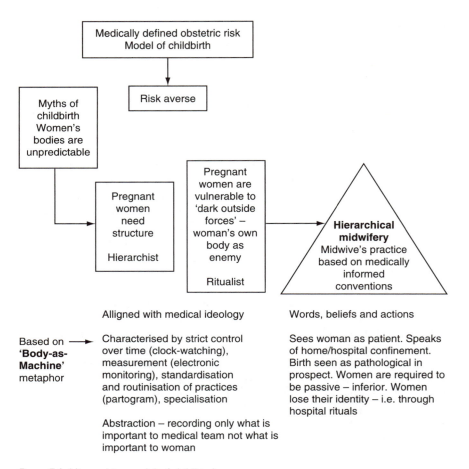

Figure 7.1 Hierarchist model of childbirth

model of maternal and child health, which leads to an ever increasing expenditure on technological development and further medicalisation. The risk concept in this case has severe limitations and yet, it continues to be used. The
simplistic quantitative concept leads to reductionist approaches and focuses
upon false risk factors, for example, grand multiparity that is a risk only in
situations of poverty (Bergstrom, 1996).

The risk model is most ardently argued in the heated debates surrounding
birth location. Many obstetricians and paediatricians argue that hospital is
the safest place for a woman to be delivered of her baby (see for example,
Campbell and Macfarlane, 1994; Chamberlain *et al.*, 1997; Davies *et al.*,
1996; Drife, 1999; Northern Region Perinatal Collaborative Survey 1996;
Young and Drife, 1992; Young and Hey, 2000). In the recent National

Sentinel Caesarean Section Audit Report (Thomas and Paranjothy, 2001), when asked to express a view about childbirth in general most women (63 per cent) agreed with the statement that 'giving birth is a natural process that should not be interfered with unless necessary'. Nearly all women strongly agreed that they would like a birth that is the safest option for their baby.

Tara's story

Tara is the thirty-something mother of Tommy. She is expecting her second child.

I had a bad time with Tommy. The pregnancy was difficult – being sick all through it and I was frightened that something would go wrong with the birth. I wanted to be in the safest place to give birth – that's the hospital. I couldn't risk my baby this time either because I am not having anymore after this so he's got to be all right. When you think of all the things that can go wrong – it doesn't seem worth taking the risk.

(Tara, England, 2000)

A small percentage (5.3) of women (3 per cent with no previous medical intervention) expressed a preference for caesarean section. These women were more likely to place a high priority on their own safety and being as free from pain as possible. They were also more likely to disagree with the statement that birth was a natural process that should not be interfered with unless necessary and agree with women's right to choose to a have a caesarean section under any circumstances. Obstetricians' opinions are given high value by women and their partners and their influence on women's 'choice' of birth is of significance here. If 51 per cent of obstetricians believe that caesarean section is the safest option for the baby and between 7 and 46 per cent of doctors would choose a caesarean themselves (Barrett et al., 1990; Guillemette and Fraser 1992; McGurgan et al., 2001), the effect upon women's choices will be profound. In the national audit referred to above, it was found that half of the obstetricians would agree to do a caesarean section in the absence of any medical intervention, if this was requested by the woman (Thomas and Paranjothy 2001). The choice obstetricians would make for themselves is in stark contrast to that of midwives and women in general. Only 4 per cent of midwives (Mitler et al., 2000) and 5 per cent of women would choose a caesarean section (Jackson and Irvine, 1998).

The global phenomenon of an increasing caesarean section rate (CSR) has been a public health concern for over 30 years and although, the timing and rate of increase has differed between countries, marked differences in rates persist. WHO (1985) issued a consensus statement suggesting there were no additional health benefits associated with a CSR above 10–15 per cent based on an examination of estimates of national caesarean section and maternal and perinatal mortality rates from various countries (Thomas and Paranjothy, ibid.).

The greatest increase in the CSR in England was seen in the 1970s when rates doubled from 4 per cent in 1970 to 9 per cent in 1980. While the increase was less marked during the 1980s, rates appeared to almost double again during the 1990s, with estimated rates of 16 per cent in 1995, and 19 per cent by 1999. Currently the CSR has risen further to 21.5 percent. According to the audit (Thomas and Paranjothy, ibid.), 20 per cent of caesarean sections are performed for failure to progress. While there was no discussion or explanation offered as to why women in the UK seemed incapable of 'normal' progress in their labours, the clock, that is, our culturally determined notions of how long a labour should last, may be an important factor. Evidence from some recent obstetric literature suggests that the problem of failure to progress may well lay with obstetric definitions of progress.

> A rate of 1 cm/hour in the active phase of labour (as in the partogram) is often accepted as the cut-off between normal and abnormal labour. The validity of this cut-off point can certainly be challenged. Too much reliance on partograms, and especially on strict protocols of action related to partogram patterns, can be an agent for regimenting labour rather than for caring for women in labour. Decisions about curtailing the second stage of labour should be based on the same principles of monitoring the wellbeing of the mother and baby that apply during the first stage of labour. If the mother's condition is satisfactory, the baby's condition is satisfactory, and there is evidence that progress is occurring with descent of the presenting part, there are no grounds for intervention.
>
> (Enkin *et al.*, 2000)

Timing and convenience are also factors in induction of labour rate, which currently stands at over 21 per cent (Department of Health, 2002). Data from the United States Centers for Disease Control show an induction rate increase from around 10 per cent to 20 per cent in the last decade with a concomitant sharp increase in induction during Monday to Friday. In the UK, earlier research has shown similar evidence of the convenience factor in induction of labour (Macfarlane, 1984) and more latterly, caesarean section (Thomas and Paranjothy, 2001) where 31 per cent of caesareans were timed to suit the mother and the staff.

The audit report highlighted the importance of one-to-one midwifery care in lowering the CSR, which must also be true for all instrumental deliveries. While 97 per cent of midwifery managers aim to provide one-on-one support in labour, only 19 per cent according to the audit report evaluated whether this level was achieved and only 50 per cent of units have sufficient midwives on the maternity suite for 94 per cent of the time. There are significant shortages of midwives. For example, the following story highlights some of the issues that arise.

Paige's story

Paige is a thirty-five-year-old woman living in a major city in the UK. She is now 36 weeks pregnant with her second child and has pre-eclampsia.

I was told that my maternity unit was closed to deliveries three times last week and I was worried that I wouldn't be able to deliver there. My blood pressure has been rising and the doctor said that I would need a caesarean section. But when they were ready to do the caesarean, the hospital's special care baby unit was closed to admissions, so I had to be moved to another hospital for my delivery. I didn't know anyone there and it was really strange – more like an airport than a hospital. I was admitted to the antenatal ward and there was another woman who had come in just before me. Her waters broke as she was walking about and she rang for the midwife who rushed in, saw what was happening, and went away again. When she came back the midwife threw incontinence pads at her and suggested that she mop up the mess herself. I was shocked but the midwife was the only person on duty in the ward and I guess she was doing the best she could.

(Paige, London, 2001)

In two randomised controlled trials in Scotland comparing midwifery care with care involving medical practitioners (Hundley *et al.*, 1994; Wagner, 1998) while there was an uneven reduction in interventions, there was more reduction in intervention in those in which there was less physician control.

Reconstructing relative risks

It is clear from research that elective caesarean sections pose greater risks to women and their babies in the short- and long-term and in future pregnancies than vaginal births do. Most of the risks obstetricians associate with vaginal birth are not inherent in the actual birth but in its management. For example, in applying time constraints associated with the onset and progress of first and second stages of labour, induction, pharmacological augmentation, epidural analgesia, episiotomy, operative vaginal delivery, and so on, labour and vaginal delivery becomes more complex and dangerous.

Childbearing may well be physically risky, but it is also a highly emotional event imbued with pleasure and joy, anxiety and pain. The motives for having (or not having) a child at a given time are changeable, contextual, and often contradictory. Having a child is a social event of great significance to immediate families, extended kin groups, communities, and other social networks. Do we really know how women in different circumstances weigh these alternatives?

For egalitarians, the application of formalised risk assessment, as a basis for making decisions about health care, is too narrow. Moreover, applying group risks to predict individual outcomes can be misleading. In 1985, a WHO report highlighted the potential of obstetric intervention to trigger a cascade of interventions. We need to listen more closely to how women in different circumstances assess the costs and benefits of alternative childbearing options, because when we recommend that a woman use obstetric care, we are asking her to take risks that we cannot predict. These include not only physical risks, but also social and emotional risks that directly concern her in a multitude of ways unknown to the obstetrician or midwife, who inhabit a very different social world.

Why did childbirth have to change?: one woman's experience

Becky's story

Becky was a seventeen-year-old woman having her first baby. She found herself in a hospital in 1999 where the policies and procedures of the institution were far more important than her needs and desires. While the midwives were being kindly and relatively friendly, to Becky's viewpoint they were distant and uncaring. In many ways Becky could be deemed fortunate since she at least had the attention of one key midwife throughout her labour. For many women this is not the case and they might be attended by a number of midwives throughout the duration of their labour and deliveries as well as other medical personnel.

Three days previously, believing herself to be in labour, Becky had gone to the local hospital only to be told that she was not in labour but just having Braxton Hicks contractions. The next evening she rang me at home to ask what she should do – she was still having contractions but was afraid to go to the hospital again. She felt they had laughed at her for her ignorance.

Two days after the birth of her baby boy in December 1999, Becky told me the story of her birth.

I was home alone because Mum had gone to work – she works in a nursing home on night duty and the baby's father was out of the picture – he'd run off months ago. I'd had the pains for a few days but they had gotten worse so I rang a friend for advice. I couldn't ring the midwife again. I'm sure she was fed up of me. Anyway we'd decided that I should go to the hospital. I called a cab and arrived in the admission room door around 2 a.m. I rang the bell as the nurse in the clinic had told me to do and the midwife opened the door and invited me in. She took my card and took me round to the admission room. The sister came round from the labour ward to see what was happening. She put her hand on my tummy and told the midwife to carry on with the admission – 'have you had your bowels opened today?' she asked – what a question to ask – I was embarrassed and didn't answer straight away – then shook my head. 'Give her an enema then, we don't want you making a mess when the baby is born do we?' What did she mean – make a mess?

It must be noted here that whilst research evidence has pointed to the redundancy of giving an enema, and many practitioners and maternity units have abandoned this practice, it appears that in one unit at least, enemas may still be in use as evidenced by Becky's reported experience and supported by midwife participants reports.

Anyway I had the enema then had to have a bath. I had only had a shower before I came out and I told the midwife but she insisted that I have another wash. I then had to dress in this awful white hospital gown which was open at the back – everyone could see my bottom. Why did I have to wear that? I told the midwife that I had brought my own nightie. 'It'll only get dirty so you might as well use ours,' she said. When I was ready, the midwife made me get on the table and started to prod my tummy. Then she put this big belt around my middle and put a cold round thing on some clips on the belt [the transducer]. She didn't tell me what she was doing. Then there was this loud thudding noise coming from the machine by the bed. 'That sounds fine' the midwife said and left the room. That must be the baby's heart, I thought.

The midwife came back and looked at the strip of paper coming out of the machine. 'I'm going to examine you now', she said. She pulled the sheet away from my legs – I was naked. She took a pack off the shelf, washed her hands and then put on some gloves. She then told me to open my legs and put my heels together. She then put her fingers inside me. Well it hurt a lot – especially since I was having a contraction at the time – it brought tears to my eyes. 'What is the matter?' the midwife asked. She was trying to be kind but she didn't stop her examination. Without telling me what she was doing, the midwife took a long pointed stick and put it into me and I felt a pop and then warm fluid running down onto the bed. [The midwife had ruptured Becky's amniotic membranes.] A few minutes later the contractions became much stronger and more painful. I was very distressed and the midwife called the doctor. 'She needs an epidural' she said. The doctor rang the anaesthetist who finally came about an hour later. 'I'm just going to put a needle in your arm and then give you a small injection in your back – you won't feel anything after that.' I hadn't asked for an epidural and they didn't tell me what effect it might have. I didn't say anything – I thought, they must know what they are doing.

Later, the contractions seemed to go off, although I couldn't tell any more so I had to have something to speed them up again. By now it was about 11a.m. and I had been left alone in the labour ward for hours – with the midwife just popping in from time to time to look at the machine or take my blood pressure. I asked if anyone had rung my mum – they hadn't of course. They didn't seem to care really.

(Becky, England, 1999)

Midwives in the United Kingdom proudly announce that they are 'with woman'. Midwives are 'with woman' when induction of labour is performed; do they question the reason? Midwives are 'with woman' when unnecessary vaginal examinations are carried out; when early amniotomies are performed to stimulate stronger contractions. Midwives are 'with woman' when fetal monitoring immobilises women into physical inactivity and psychological passivity; when systemic analgesics are used inappropriately; when women are coached in second stage to 'push, push, don't waste the push'; and so on. Do midwives who are 'with woman' seek to restore to the woman the authority for her own body – authority that has been eroded over generations? Or do they stand by passively as the labouring woman progressively loses confidence in her ability to birth, then nod their heads sympathetically when she says she needs an epidural?

Becky had been defined as high risk in this context because she was seventeen, unmarried, and did not appear to be well educated – an assumption based perhaps on the fact that she failed to answer questions quickly and that she cried when examined. The power differential in this case was clearly in the favour of the midwife and doctors who attended Becky. She had little say in determining the course of her own labour. Many would argue that the pain of childbirth only becomes intolerable when a woman is in hospital, removed from her own environment and where her ability to exert control over the events diminishes (Symonds and Hunt, 1996: 94). Arney (1982) argued that pain relief is itself a way of exercising control over women. Moreover, an epidural renders a woman not only powerless but also immobile in more ways than one (as discussed in chapter 6). The pain of humiliation is as great for some women as the pain of childbirth and indeed, may well exacerbate it. This in turn renders the woman dependent upon the midwives and medical staff. The culture of dependency ensures that the doctor who is the expert makes the really important decisions. So Becky's birth becomes pathological, an illness requiring diagnosis and medical intervention to ensure a safe outcome. As Illich (1976) stated, 'Diagnosis always intensifies stress, defines incapacity, imposes inactivity, and focuses apprehension on non-recovery, on uncertainty, and on one's dependence on future medical findings, all of which amounts to a loss of autonomy or self-definition.' When pregnancy and labour become a matter of diagnostic concern, then women are automatically constrained within that framework. It must be remembered though that women over generations have been inculcated into the view that childbirth is risky, that doctors are the culture heroes who can 'fix' their problems and that hospitals are the safest place for themselves and their babies. The media, popular television and film have been vehicles by which this message has been transmitted.

Striving for egalitarianism

In 1976 two student midwives shared their frustration and disappointment with the increasing medicalisation and intervention in maternity care and began meeting regularly for mutual support and study. Others joined them and in 1978 the group named themselves the Radical Midwives.

In the mid 1970s, a large number of pregnant women in UK had labour induced by artificial rupture of membranes (ARM) around the date they were 'due'. These initials were in use when the group needed a name, and so the Association of Radical Midwives was established, using the dictionary definition of 'radical', (roots, origins, basics, etc.) which aptly described the basic midwifery skills they hoped to revive.

By the early 1980s, childbirth was already beginning to change. Both women and midwives, influenced by reading literature and from experiences of birth in different contexts in different countries, began to practise alternative approaches to childbirth that challenged the dominant medical model. These women and practitioners aligned themselves with a cultural type that viewed women's bodies as robust and birth as a natural, everyday occurrence. They adopted a social, egalitarian model of childbirth (see figure 7.2) that enhanced the social aspects of childbirth as well as ensuring the safety aspects were addressed. Birth was defined as physiological. The woman was seen as the active and powerful central player in the birth event. The language is one of the social rather than medical world. In this model women maintain their identity and their control.

Kate's story

Kate was a woman in her mid-thirties who was having her first baby. She had read extensively and was a member of the National Childbirth Trust. She was committed to having an active birth after hearing Janet Balakas speak at a conference. Kate's husband was fully supportive that this labour should be drug free and as active as possible with Kate walking around the room unencumbered by technology.

It must have looked a strange sight. Here, amongst some of the world's most advanced obstetric technology Kate was giving birth on the floor.

Kate was not from some foreign land, she was just an English woman who had read about and wanted an active birth. She had arrived at the hospital in

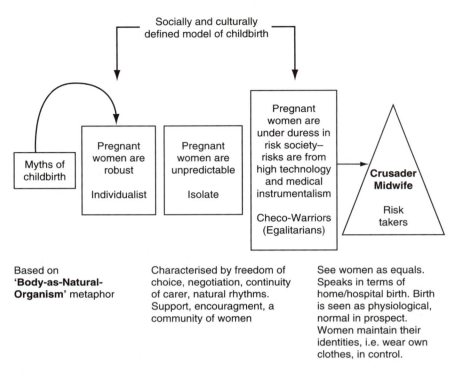

Figure 7.2 Egalitarian model of childbirth

advanced labour and while the midwife was reviewing her antenatal records, Kate had quietly left her bed and began squatting on the floor. As she squatted, her waters broke. The midwife hurriedly placed some 'sterile' sheets under her and joined her in a squatting position. Within minutes, a healthy baby girl slipped gently into the hands of the midwife. I was that midwife and this was more than fifteen years ago long before Changing Childbirth.

(Midwife's birth report, England, 1985)

The anomalous image of a squatting woman giving birth surrounded by the gleaming, modern equipment in a labour ward is a fitting metaphor for the problematic relationship some midwives have with technology. The question is can midwifery, with its low-technology, non-intervention tradition, find a place in an environment where competence is equated with the use of the latest, high-technology procedures? In deciding how to respond to the new technologies of birth, midwives face a dilemma: if they adopt the instruments of modern medicine, they risk sacrificing their distinctive tradition; if they cling to their tradition, they risk marginalisation as old-fashioned, bizarre, or perhaps, even dangerous practitioners. The dilemma of 'midwives among the machines', is also, in fact, a problem for women in childbirth in the United Kingdom as elsewhere. As the world around them changes, women and midwives must adapt, they must 'recreate' themselves.

The beginnings of change

Left in the hands of medical practitioners and their strong government lobby, costs of maternity services escalated because of the assumptions made that more obstetric care and intervention would mean less death and morbidity. This was and continues to be aided and abetted by the media and the legal system. As British society becomes increasingly litigious, any hope for less medical intervention and its consequent high expenditure and more social amelioration of health hazards will decline. Nevertheless, growing concerns regarding the costs of maternity care in the 1980s spawned a number of studies (Annandale, 1989; Clark, Mugford, and Mugford, 1990; 1993; Romalis, 1981) which were beginning to show that centralisation of maternity units was not based on good evidence about the cost-effectiveness of the policy. Furthermore, research found that the outcome for women in terms of satisfaction and infant and maternal morbidity appeared to be no worse in midwife run schemes than obstetric schemes and might even be improved (Flint *et al.*, 1989). Reviews of the evidence on place of birth suggested that planned home birth for women with low obstetric risk had similar (Campbell and Macfarlane, 1987) or even better outcomes (Tew, 1985; 1990) than those of a woman equally at low risk, giving birth in hospital.

The changing experience of women

Beverly's story

Beverly is a middle-class, well-educated woman in her mid-thirties, having her second child.

I was kneeling on the floor in the labour ward. It was the most comfortable position to relieve my backache. The midwife entered the room and immediately got down beside me. 'Would you like to deliver in this position?' she asked. 'If you do then I will organise a clean field on which to deliver your baby.' I had not thought of doing that – I told the midwife that I was happy to hop up onto the bed if that was more convenient for her. 'No,' she said, she was happy to deliver me in any position I chose. I was quite surprised that the midwife asked if I wanted to deliver on the floor. I had had a baby not two years previously in this very hospital and that was not the attitude then. At that time I had to conform to the hospital policy and deliver on my back – well, half-reclining on the bed. I wondered what had changed. Of course, I was having my first child then and I supposed that had made a difference. I was better prepared this time – having been through it before and so was more confident in myself and knew what I wanted. Perhaps that confidence made a difference to the staff. Anyway, the midwife stayed with me throughout the labour, some five hours, popping in and out but never away too long. I felt comfortable with her and the birth was comparatively easy. Emily, my daughter was born with me kneeling on the floor. After it was all over, I suddenly realised that I had not needed any pain relief – I felt wonderful – awake and alert unlike the last time!

(Beverly, England, 1999)

Beverly appears to have had a satisfying experience and was indeed happy with the outcome of the birth. Perhaps it would be interesting to assess why she had such a response for if we go back to Becky's story, one can see a significant difference in approach. Clearly, Beverly had the advantage of being an articulate, well-educated middle-class woman. She was indeed fortunate to have a midwife who could devote sufficient time to her to ensure she had a satisfying and safe birth. For many women and midwives this may not be the case with the growing crisis in midwifery as a result of staff shortages.

Before we all congratulate ourselves on how bad doctors are and how midwives can save the childbearing world, let's be honest about the state of the profession. We consider ourselves the guardians of normal childbirth but that is becoming less of a fact, with the numbers of midwives as sole carer dropping all the time. The reality is that, on the whole, midwives are exhausted and fed up. The constant struggle of working on labour wards staffed by four midwives at a time coping with shifts that usually have at least two epidurals and then the inevitable caesarean section, water births, premature labours, terminations, high-dependency care of eclampsia, etc., etc., are taking their toll. Many midwives now have more skills than junior doctors and are expected to undertake all these tasks as well as being with women.

(Schan, 1998)

Symbolic exchanges: recreating childbirth and midwifery

The sources of change in the context of childbirth and midwifery practice are varied. The need for midwifery 're-creation' is often the result of change coming from within the profession itself. As the health industry develops new technology and new techniques, midwives among other practitioners must adapt, changing practices and discarding old theories, making room for the latest professional information. Change in technology, however, is only one source of change originating within or outside midwifery. Decisions regarding the organisation of midwifery also bring about change. As midwifery develops new educational programmes, creates new areas of specialisation, or reallocates tasks among other occupational groups, the profession reformulates itself. These same processes can also set in motion a course of action that results in unintended, sometimes negative, consequences for childbearing women and midwives as the following comment from one frustrated midwife shows.

> In my unit we have reduced the use of Pethidine down to about 3 per cent of women, but it is very difficult to persuade women and midwives that alternatives such as massage and support will work when it is impossible to provide one-to-one care. Community midwives fare no better – 24 hours on call at a time – which can involve a full day of visits and clinics and in our area up to two or three times in the night to home births or helping on labour ward. This is a service run on goodwill and loyalty.
>
> (Schan, 1998)

Societal and cultural changes are important sources of professional re-creation. Included among the many influences exerted on medicine by society, for example, are changes in the local, national and global economy that may drive the reorganisation of health care financing. Changes in the political environment and demographic shifts such as baby booms, ageing populations, and increased urbanisation all present challenges to the way that institutions and individual practitioners organise themselves. Health care systems must also adjust to shifts in cultural concerns regarding gender, family, work, science, and religion. For example, health care changed in response to developing cultural conceptions of gender. The gender balance in medical occupations has also changed, though what this may mean for women in childbirth is still unknown.

A profession's history and consequent cultural authority determine the freedom it has to shape its place in the medical marketplace. Professions with greater prestige, greater income, and greater power are freer to influence political, organisational, and cultural processes. Professions like nursing, established as an adjunct to the profession of physicians, find their position controlled by those with more 'social capital'. Professions closely connected to a tradition, like midwifery and homeopathy, find their ability to adjust and recreate themselves limited by that tradition. In the following pages, the ways in which midwifery is attempting to recreate itself is examined. First the factors that influence, enhance and impede the midwives' task of recreating themselves, are examined. Next the strategies of re-creation used by midwives on both organisational and individual levels are explored using data from fieldwork in England to highlight the socially situated nature of professional re-creation.

Strategies of re-creation

The changed cultural attitudes of the 1960s and the economic realities of the 1980s and 1990s allowed midwives in Britain to maintain a foothold in modern medical systems. But the future of the profession remains unclear. To the extent that it promises to manage risk and to reduce pain, the machinery of modern obstetrics has wide appeal. Midwives face the difficult task of finding a way of recreating midwifery that preserves the distinctiveness of the profession while remaining up-to-date in obstetric techniques.

The strategies used by midwives to respond to this unmanageable situation fall into two categories:

- organisational strategies: efforts undertaken by, or on behalf of, midwife organisations to preserve a place for the midwifery profession in the medical marketplace; and
- individual strategies, efforts undertaken by individual midwives to establish and protect the distinct practice of midwifery. These strategies of re-creation, be they organisational or individual, are influenced by the social context, a fact that is apparent in the contrast between the situations of midwives in the United Kingdom, the United States, Ghana, Malawi and Malaysia.

The 'assimilationist' strategy of re-creation

The 'assimilationist' strategy of re-creation chosen by some midwives threatened to extinguish the separate tradition of midwifery. In effect, midwives were exchanging their own tradition for the tradition of medicine or nursing. Societal and cultural change in the form of the feminist movement and a new and vigorous questioning of technology gave midwives the opportunity to emphasise their distinct tradition, to recreate themselves as separate from medicine.

In the light of this new cultural atmosphere midwives attempted to renew their identity as a 'low-tech, high-touch', women-centred occupation. The very image that weakened the profession earlier in the century now gave them a niche in the medical marketplace. Midwives found further support for their profession extending their appeal beyond new cultural ideas about women and technology to economic concerns of policy makers and health care administrators. But this has backfired as the following midwife's comments highlight:

Almost a decade has passed since the publication of 'Changing Childbirth'

(1993). And the question must be asked – are midwives better off? Are women better off? Many would say 'No'. Changing Childbirth was the great hope for turning the tide back to midwifery-led care and empowerment for all, but the reality is rising Caesarean section and epidural rates and decreasing numbers of babies being delivered by midwives (ENB, 1997). There seem to be pockets of excellence reported all over the country, yet a normal delivery, i.e. a birth without any intervention, becomes increasingly unusual. Midwives have begun to congratulate each other for 'getting a normal delivery'!

(Schan, 1998)

If we are honest, maternity services on the whole are in disarray – underfunded and overstretched, being held together by tired and demoralised midwives who feel dispensable and undervalued. The knowledge and skills of midwives are recognised within our profession, but are barely acknowledged by the people with real power – the obstetric hierarchy and the media. These are the people that women listen to and are influenced by. How can we change a whole generation which now consider technological birth to be the norm and are grateful when the doctors step in to 'save' them? Elective caesarean sections and epidurals are sold to women as the ultimate informed choice for the feminist, yet I consider having the birth of your baby controlled by machines and conducted by an unknown man (or woman) in an operating theatre the epitome of disempowerment (Schan, 1998).

Increasingly there is an emphasis given to a more holistic problem solving approach (Feuerstein, 1993; Pansini-Murrell, 1996; Thomas, et al., 1998; Thomas and Cooke, 1999) to midwifery practice and education based on a systematic assessment of biological, psychological and social needs. This has led to the need to understand pregnancy and birth from these various perspectives which in turn means that midwives need to draw from the behavioural and social sciences those concepts and theories pertinent to the care they seek to deliver. Yet we are probably failing in achieving the stated goals. Ultimately, the approach midwives take to childbirth is determined by their cultural alignment, both in terms of their own sociocultural, ethnic or religious group and in terms of their beliefs and values concerning childbirth and midwifery practice (see figures 7.1 and 7.2). For some it is a matter of survival, others rebel and either leave the profession or crusade against what they see as the 'immorality' of medical practice. Still others simply assimilate to the local cultural environment.

For midwives working in the community setting, their cultural alignment may be determined by the culture in which they live and work. It is only in the context of the hospital where midwives are separated from the social context of childbirth, that midwives may develop a 'midwifery culture'.

In the United Kingdom, fieldwork revealed the general dichotomy held by midwives about the fragility-robustness of pregnant women. Many argued that pregnancy was normal and natural, but midwives had to watch and examine women to ensure that pregnancy stayed that way, thus revealing an underlying fear that pregnancy is not normal or robust, that women need structure and are unpredictable. Some activists in the United Kingdom would argue that pregnant women are under duress. In Douglas's (1997) terms this would be taken to mean that childbearing women's bodies are fragile and pregnancy can be lethal. Such a view would justify the fears and anxieties of obstetricians and midwives. Indeed, women have been socialised into this view in the Western world. However, I would argue that for some, the view of duress would be in terms of the risk posed by modern society to women in childbirth. I have given the name checo-warriors (childbirth ecology warriors) to the political activists who attempt to challenge and change modern technological concepts of childbirth.

Another view of duress was found among experienced midwives in a focus group discussion about childbirth. Most of the midwives had children in their late teens and twenties. The majority had studied midwifery in the 1970s. They claimed to have been influenced by teachers such as Lamaze, Leboyer, Kitzinger, and more recently Odent, Wagner, Flint, Leap and many others.

The midwives were each committed to effecting change in their profession and demedicalising pregnancy and childbirth. One was a leader in the home-birth movement; she was confident after many years of independent practice. Another had worked in Africa and so had experienced a different approach to maternity care. Another worked in a country hospital. Four midwives were part of a group midwifery practice attached to a local private hospital under the 'protection' of a group of obstetricians. Some had been leaders in the profession and were in private practice. Two were managers of maternity units, seeking to implement new models of midwifery care into the system.

They viewed women as being under duress if they had social problems, consequently, while women may not 'need' doctors, they certainly needed midwives who would guide them through their pregnancies, giving advice and identifying abnormalities as they arose. The predominant cultural type that emerged among the research participants was that of the hierarchist –'women need structure', to justify midwives' own controls and planned projects. For many women, they were quite content to fall into the structural category during pregnancy although they might adopt a different cultural type in other areas of their lives.

Even pregnant midwives still conform to the hierarchist cultural type. Despite their own knowledge base, they look to the institutions to offer structure and control which may ultimately mean that they believe that women's bodies in pregnancy are unpredictable. Instead of becoming isolated they cling ever more strongly to the hierarchical model for security. Obstetricians on the other hand fall mainly into the category which views women's bodies as fragile and pregnancy as dangerous in an effort to justify their own anxieties and fears. From this stance such mechanisms as automatic induction of labour in prolonged pregnancy, routine electronic fetal monitoring despite the evidence of its low value, and starvation during labour in case the woman needs a general anaesthetic brings a feeling of security for obstetricians, regardless of research evidence to the contrary. All women are treated in exactly the same way so that the doctors can be assured that their controls have been implemented.

Haven't we all experienced the intrusion of ultrasound and other forms of prenatal testing into pregnancy? 'Quickening', (the time when a woman first feels the movements of her baby), is no longer an important date to remember. The black and white flickering screen of the ultrasound shows not only movement but also a heartbeat, and that is often prior to quickening. The woman can take home pictures, even videos, far more concrete than that small fluttering feeling.

(Jane, 1998)

I've participated in continuous fetal monitoring, when the woman was no longer the focus of attention. The piece of paper rolling out of the machine and the sounds picked up by the transducer were what everyone, including the woman herself, paid attention to. Women used to be able to walk about, ignoring outside interference – these patterns of behaviour, which helped the progress of labour, are now over-taken by the fascination with technology.

(Beth, 1998)

Drugs and epidurals also block the woman's natural pain relieving agents – her production of endorphins. It was no wonder that we have seen rising rates of operative childbirth. By the time the decision is made to take the baby [out] by forceps or caesarean section, the woman is thanking the good doctor for rescuing her and her baby from their dreadful state. Technology has replaced touch. Machinery has minimised the value of a woman's role in this essentially female experience.

(Mary, 1998)

I can understand why midwives are looking for something better, whether they work in hospitals or in the community. I find it difficult to understand why more midwives don't question the system, don't feel dissatisfied with the excessive imposition of medical technology into the birthing processes of well women.

(Clare, 1998)

The midwives in this study displayed a perspective adhering to one of four cultural types – that women's bodies are robust. The question must be asked – what makes these midwives different from other more conventional midwives?

In the United Kingdom the battle lines remain drawn between those who support a hundred per cent hospital, medically controlled delivery and those who support home birth as a safe option for low-risk women. The battle was never simply between midwives and medical men. It was much more complex than that. The battle is between differing and opposing cultural types.

If we take Mary Douglas' (1997: 22) theory of myths of persons, with a little ingenuity we can turn this cultural analysis around so as to apply it to childbirth. In the contest about childbirth, the threat of infinite regress is blocked by reference to the nature of the childbearing woman's body. The choices relate to regulation and control.

Whoever wants to claim that pregnant women's bodies are robust enough to give birth without intervention is using that argument to defend the entrepreneur's claim to conduct birth as she feels is appropriate – without constraints. We would expect that claim to be reversed in the case of the person on whom that obstetrician or midwife or indeed, a woman, wishes to put constraints. The individualist/entrepreneur practitioner or pregnant woman will claim that women's bodies are robust so long as they are not put under stifling controls; women's bodies need to be free and will suffer damage if controlled.

The isolate, with no reason for sustaining any particular view of childbirth, maintains an uninvolved eclecticism. Meanwhile, the hierarchist, whose way of life is to organise and be organised, and whose justification is that women's bodies can only be safe if they are regulated, will argue that it is the nature of women to thrive in organisations. Structure is a necessary support for childbirth.

In the light of the changes in attitude, midwives attempted to re-establish their professional identity as 'low tech, high touch', women-centred practitioners. Childbearing women's bodies are seen as vulnerable and pregnancy can be lethal as a result of societal and environmental risk. This position is entered in fundamental disagreement with the policies of the individualists and with organising hierarchists, and with the fatalism of the isolate. It justifies political activism on behalf of women to redress the balance of society and nature. This lifestyle focuses on activating the community to effect change in the social conditions of the individual and the individual's role in contesting risk challenges.

To take the analogy further, from my studies I have identified another cultural type – perhaps not strictly of the same order as those identified by Douglas (1997), but relevant to the case in hand, that is – the ritualist. In this permutation, ritualists fear not following rules and rituals regardless of evidence put before them, for fear of unleashing unforeseen dark and mysterious forces – this is the just in case syndrome. Most modern midwives and obstetricians would not admit to belonging to such a group, but the evidence from the narratives and observations is indicative of their cultural alignment, even if their discourse was different.

The source of foundation myths of nature also produce foundational models of persons and models of childbirth, justifying or rejecting claims of authority from other persons (Douglas, 1997: 22). If these four cultural types of childbirth are sound they deliver the practitioner and pregnant woman from the reproach of superficial fashion-proneness in childbirth choices. It is a cultural competition that causes the underlying coherence of childbirth consumption choices. Cultural competition is a matter of conscience. Looking for coherence from the point of view of individual psychology will never reveal the conscientious woman, midwife or obstetrician defending a cultural outpost. Psychology has no idea of what they might be protesting against. But according to cultural theory, when they choose a method of childbirth they choose a flag to wave and they know whom they are waving it against. Childbirth is a public show – to encourage fainthearted followers the woman, midwife or obstetrician may want to stay loyal and deliver in hospital or break out and have the baby at home. Either way, the place of birth is a sign – a symbol of cultural alignment. The choices are acts of defiance, intimidation and persuasion. Having a baby at home is wielding a weapon – the home is a badge of allegiance; just as modern technology in the form of the electronic fetal monitor is a badge of allegiance. Choosing the tools and approaches to birth is declaring dogma. Childbirth demands constant attention. Pressed hard by enemy forces, it calls for constant vigilance, subtlety and resourcefulness.

Conclusion

There are persistent calls from women, pressure groups and midwives for a balance between considerations for the safety and the social aspects of childbirth. Women in the UK do not need to be under the care of an obstetrician during their pregnancy or childbirth. Despite the apparent greater freedom of choice women have in the UK, there remains dissatisfaction among both women and midwives.

Over the past two decades, childbirth began to change but in two diametrically opposed directions. One is towards woman-centred, holistic care provided by midwives, and the other is towards increasingly high-technology obstetric management. In an attempt to mediate across the divide, midwives, women and obstetricians have more or less adopted a risk approach to childbirth. Obstetricians have used risk assessment to identify women who may have major medical difficulties during pregnancy or delivery.

Meanwhile, reviews of the evidence on place of birth suggested that planned home birth for women with low obstetric risk had similar or better outcomes than those of women equally at low risk, giving birth in hospital. Over time articulate middle-class women and midwives, influenced by reading literature and from experiences of birth in different contexts in different countries, began to influence childbirth practice by engaging in alternative

Chapter 8

Symbolic exchanges in childbirth

Reflections from the case studies

> The forces of modernity have taken childbirth away from the realm of social life and placed it into the professional health arena.
>
> (Jarvis, 2000, in conversation)

It is often the people living ordinary lives far removed from the corridors of power who have the clearest perception of what is really happening. Yet they are often reluctant to speak openly of what they believe in their hearts to be true. It is too frightening and too different from what those with more impressive credentials and access to the media are saying. Their suppressed insights may leave them feeling isolated and helpless (Korten, 1995).

The purpose of this chapter is to attempt to draw together the threads of women's experiences of childbirth in the case studies chapters and explore the complexities, contradictions and consequences of globalisation for women in childbirth and those who attend them. This analysis, drawing upon some of the concerns and strategies of feminist cultural studies, seeks to illuminate how linguistic processes intersect with social structures, professional authority, economic resources, and political activism to produce gendered representations of social life and specifically of childbirth and women's health. Its ultimate aim is to propose a more complex theoretical understanding of how definitions of childbirth come to be constructed, codified, and mobilised. This in turn seems an essential prerequisite for developing more intelligent childbirth policies and practices globally.

The shape of the social world affects ways of thinking about that world. As people, we continually create our social world and are being created by it. Dichotomised sex roles, as an example, have been internalised as real by people all over the world, regardless of whether they exist 'really'. Whether sociology texts, psychotherapists, advice-to-the-lovelorn columnists, television characters, pastoral counselling, jokes or relatives and friends perpetuate the socially constructed roles, they exist and affect all of us, constructing and controlling behaviour.

Symbolic exchanges in childbirth: the influence of science and medicine

One of the key symbolic exchanges in childbirth is associated with the notion of obstetric risk. Risk is built on the technology of numbers and the ideology and practice of scientific calculation. Medicine needed quantification to acquire credibility as a science. Medicine represents a 'cultural association between the notions of professional expertise, objectivity and the impersonality states, (depersonalisation. . . .) afforded by the technology of numbers' (Oakley, 2000: 110).

Quantification, according to Oakley (ibid.: 103) is a social technology and as such it raises all the sorts of problems associated with other technologies. Technology is not value-free. It is shaped by the social and economic context that gives rise to it. It is designed to meet certain needs, but as Oakley points out these are not everyone's needs. Technology often has all sorts of unforeseen consequences in specific social contexts; some of which, are likely to damage the very goals those technologies were designed to espouse. Such is the case in the context of childbirth.

More than one hundred years ago, science and social science had come to mean the use of quantitative methods to discover the laws governing the universe. The view was taken that everything that was worth anything could be represented by a number (Thomas Hobbes 1588–1679, and John Stewart Mill).

Porter argued that numbers form an approach to communication that impose remoteness and dispassion on what would formerly have been familiar relationships.

> Most crucially, reliance on numbers and quantitative manipulation minimizes the need for intimate knowledge and personal trust. . . . Quantification is well suited for communication that goes beyond the boundaries of locality and community. A highly disciplined discourse helps to produce knowledge independent of the particular people who make it.
>
> (Porter, 1995: ix)

If this is taken in conjunction with the rise of professionalisation and specialisation in modern society, this creates a situation in which expertise is inseparable from objectivity. This in turn, according to Oakley (2000: 113), allows objectivity to be aligned with the reduction of everything to numbers. Equally there is a conceptual link to the idea of validity. Consequently the most valid knowledge is produced, or described, by using numbers. Oakley points out that the Latin root of 'validity' means 'power'. Power, therefore, is derived from knowledge expressed numerically and those most powerful are in a position to know better, or more, than others are.

The emphasis on precision created the frame of mind, which made the inventions of the Industrial Revolution possible. The growth of abstract numerical calculations is a feature of an increasingly complex society.

(Oakley, 2000: 113)

When coupled with the social regulation of time, the rise of quantification became part of a professional move towards standardised rules that could be communicated between people, across continents, thereby diminishing the human element in knowledge production. In medicine, this process served to impose a distance between practitioners and their patients. The increase in mechanical and electronic ways of knowing what is happening inside a person's body obviates the need for that person to tell doctors what they think and feel is happening to them.

Medical technologically produced information about the body has a numerical form. For example, the ultrasonic scan produces a picture of the fetus along with measurements of its size; the electronic monitor churns out computer printouts of the speed of the fetal heart rate, and the strength and length of uterine contractions. Midwives using their hands to estimate the strength and length of uterine contraction or to listen to the fetal heart using a fetal stethoscope did not provide 'objective' data for anyone else to hear or feel or challenge. The machines, like the flexible stethoscope effectively acts to create a distance between the practitioner and the woman. Oakley (2000: 115) saw this as one of the unforeseen consequences brought about by the introduction of technology.

Furthering the numerical paradigm: 'measuring' the risk of childbirth

In the modern world people are expected to live and die subject to known, measurable natural forces, not subject to mystical, mysterious moral agencies. Science wrought this change in thinking between the modern and premodern world and as Douglas and Wildavsky (1983: 49) argued, has actually expanded the universe beyond that which we can talk about with confidence. As science delves deeper into the unknown through research and investigation, Douglas and Wildavsky argue that one can assume that humankind can now be more informed about the smallest sources of danger as well as the largest. But perception of infinite risk introduces the double-edged thrust of science, generating new ignorance with new knowledge. The same ability to search out and see causes and connections between the smallest parts of the universe can leave more unexplained than was left by cruder measuring instruments. As experts disagree, they have to find more and more evidence. This results in ever-deeper analysis. But expanding measurement only increases the area of ignorance. The frustration of scientists is a characteristic feature of modern times.

The estimation of risk is a scientific question – and therefore, a legitimate activity of scientists. The acceptability of a given level of risk, however, is a political question, to be determined in the political arena. The moment there is disagreement or controversy, that is to say, when someone says a risk is unacceptable, the question becomes political. We now see that the question needs to move from establishing facts to establishing acceptability of childbirth risk, from correct answers to agreed conclusions. Inevitably we need a way of scaling the warnings and promises of science to the limited realm of political possibility. In health care generally and obstetrics in particular, one such way of making such assessment is by ascribing cost-effective measurement to risk analysis.

To accomplish this purpose, techniques of obstetric risk calculation and comparing probabilities have been developing for the last three centuries. Do the methods of obstetric risk assessment tell us what risks women face? Or does the choice of method imply a prior choice of the risks we have already chosen to face or to escape?

The political argument over obstetric technology is conducted between the heavily risk averse and the risk takers. The risk-averse side starts from the point that nature and the natural environment are unpredictable and need structure, that women's bodies are flawed and need to be monitored and controlled in order to avoid harm and that pregnancy and childbirth are pathological in prospect and only timely intervention can reverse the decline into complications and abnormality. The level of surveillance required and the technology and instrumentation needed to correct or avoid dangers exert a substantial cost. Governments and individuals need to weigh the costs in order to make decisions about the relative cost-benefits of certain obstetric activities.

The risk-takers side says that nature is good and that women's bodies are robust. Pregnancy and childbirth are normal, everyday processes and women are advised that if they trust their bodies and live a normal, healthy lifestyle, pregnancy and childbirth risk will be reduced with very little or no obstetric intervention. The risk averse will have no part in this argument. They insist that human life must be preserved at all costs and that means control and intervention. But this may not be simply a feature ·of modern society. In traditional societies in Africa and Malaysia, for example, pregnant women, traditional healers, and birth attendants practice all sorts of rituals to avoid danger or intervene when things go wrong.

Risk assessment would be easier in a settled society so certain of its values that its processes for discovering facts and making political decisions would be judged fully adequate. That would be a trusting society, but it is not the world in which we live. There is neither agreement over appropriate methods to assess childbirth risks nor acceptance of the outcomes of public processes. The problems have subjective and objective facets and risk assessment needs to deal with each.

The exercise of rational choice must include selection of focus, weighting of values, and editing of problems. But this editing process cannot be well done as a specialised exercise in thinking about risks. Specialised risk analysis impoverishes the statement of a human problem by taking it out of context. The notion of risk is an extraordinary idea, essentially decontextualised and desocialised. Thinking about how to choose between risks, subjective values must take priority. It is a travesty of rational thought to pretend that it is best to take value-free decisions in matters of life and death.

One salient difference between experts (obstetricians) and the lay public (women) is that the latter, when assessing risks, do not conceal their moral commitments but put them into the argument, explicitly and prominently. The private person does not isolate risk elements to address them directly. When she consults, she tries to consult people who understand her situation (the midwife, the TBA). This is paramount in her choice of midwife or general medical practitioner. Only when desperate does she consult the unbiased, technically superior expert (the obstetrician). Instead of submerging the risk elements in the larger pattern of social commitments, the medical expert can speak to a narrow issue beyond which professional requirements forbid him to go. The ordinary woman admits that her loyalties and moral obligations are largely the matter at stake, but the risk expert claims to depoliticise an inherently political problem.

Humans are not isolated individuals. Their sociality should be included in the analysis of how their minds work. In risk perception, humans act less as individuals and more as social beings that have internalised social pressures and delegated their decision-making processes to institutions that act as problem simplifying devises.

When pressed to give an account of a decision, the pregnant woman will refer to the experts or indeed her partner or family. She will also make a show of objective consideration of the problem. In private life as much as in public life, no one undertakes the kind of cognitive analysis that the risk assessors do when they try to separate the problem from everything except the pure calculation of probabilities. The risk assessors offer an objective analysis. We know that is not objective so long as they are dealing with uncertainties and operating on big guesses. They slide their personal bias into the calculations unobserved. The expert pretends to derive statements about what ought to be from statements about what is. The individual tends to start from ought and so does not subscribe to the ancient fallacy. If this were the difference between experts and lay people, good logic would be on the side of the latter. But the separation of 'ought' from 'is' cannot be clearly made. 'Ought' depends on what is possible. The limits of the possible depend on what is known about the conditions of physical existence. Consequently, the question of whether development ought to reduce maternal mortality has to consider what is possible under the conditions under which women are living. What is known about the conditions is small compared to what is not known – that risk assessors are not the only ones who fill the gaps in knowledge with educated guesses. The kinds of guesses made about childbirth depend very largely on the kinds of moral education of the people doing the guessing.

Everyone, expert and lay person alike, is biased. Knowledge of danger is necessarily partial and limited; judgement of risk and safety must be selected as much on the basis of what is valued as on the basis of what is known. Thus the difference diminishes between modern people and non-modern. Science and risk assessors cannot tell us what we need to know about threats of danger since they explicitly try to exclude moral ideas about the good life. Where responsibility starts, they stop.

Individuals who pass on their decision-making process to institutional processes are not washing their hands of responsibility. The responsible action is to have built good monitoring devices so that one's own friends and neighbours will defend principles. Family life and work life focus and restrict the individual vision. Careful to avoid disgrace and conscious of the need of support, the social being is a sensitive scanner of safety signs in a universe of critical fellow human beings who share her commitments. It seems that rational behaviour does not use elaborate calculation for making crisis decisions, nor does it separate out risks one by one. Rather it focuses on the infrastructure of everyday conduct, establishing the conditions for survival by building flexible, feasible aims in a way of life. Individual decisions are in a way less complicated than national decisions but the methods of simplifying are still sound. Serious risk analysis should also focus on the institutional framework of decision-making. The real choices that lead most directly to dangerous decisions are choices about social institutions. Instead of being distracted by dubious calculations, we should instead focus our analysis on what is wrong with the state of society.

To understand risk perception in the context of childbirth we should ask what makes a danger seem highly improbable when the psychologist does not provide percentages on the probabilities. We should ask how gains are ranked when there is no clear money standard on which to compare them. The current theories of risk perception steer badly between over intellectualising the decision process and over emphasising irrational impediments. It is as if the individual would reject them immediately if only she could perceive the dangers to health and safety known to the experts. This is to intellectualise the use of knowledge beyond all reason. The satisfaction in smoking and drinking, for example, are not private pleasures. Even if they were, habits would still be hard to change because they are locked into lifestyles. But most habits good and bad, are social, rooted in community life. One does not always feel free to admonish friends to change their work and leisure patterns or even to utter silent reproaches for deviation, and to withdraw from shared occasions would be asking too much. It is enough of an effort to meet the criticisms of colleagues, friends and family by coming up to their standards;

persuading them to adopt new practices decreed by health agents is quite another thing.

The issue is that anyone who lives in a community is monitored, the more close-knit, the more mutual monitoring occurs. Such monitoring constitutes the social bond. In a close community a person has often needs to work hard to meet the neighbours' standards. This is where she acquires childbirth and health education, advice and reference to experts when things appear to go wrong. When the community bond is weaker, she can relax. She can choose among her friends; but unless she is totally isolated, the acquaintances to whom she goes to for solace are her source of risk warning. A real life risk portfolio is not a selection made by private rationalisation. In real life the social process slides the decision-making and the prior editing of choices onto social institutions. Shared values do more than weight the calculations of risks. They work on the estimates of probabilities as well as on the perceived magnitude of loss.

Nothing influences the estimate of probabilities more than the sense of future time. Most people conceive time as a straight extension of the present, but there are large variations. Oscar Lewis maintained that the condition of poverty foreshortens the future. The very poor, not knowing where their next meal will come from, get the habit of living so entirely in the present that they do not imagine the future at all (Lewis, 1966).

Comparison of risk perception should allow for local conceptions of time. The official view of how to assess the future starts from the experience of time as measured by clocks and calendars and by the projections upon these measures. Everyone committed to a social life is committed to an appropriate structure of time. Deep differences in attitudes towards risk derive from institutional life and these can be traced over time. Apart from estimating a timescale for a problem of choice, even the size of a problem is differently estimated according to the cultural bias that is part of institutions for organising actions. People who have recently suffered a childbirth catastrophe are more likely to imagine it happening to them. The more distant such an experience, the more difficult to imagine oneself in that situation. The more dramatic a loss, the easier to remember it.

Some institutions keep the story of past disasters alive, while others cherish only the good ones. On assigning magnitude to a possible disaster, everything depends on which items of information are included and which ignored. So, for example, one of the functions of obstetric practice in the United Kingdom is to remind those involved of each and every maternal disaster, through a process of repeated reviews. At local level each hospital has frequent reviews of cases to consider where they went wrong and what risks they represent for other women. The statistics gathered over a three-year period from all maternity units are complied into a report and distributed widely to remind all those involved of the dangers associated with childbirth. Thus the emphasis is on pathology and complications of pregnancy and childbirth rather than on the majority of women who have 'normal' births.

General social orientations – a zero-sum or expanded-sum view of childbirth, short or long-term horizons, concentration on losses or gains – guide selection of risks. Overall goals provide the selective principles, and there is reason to believe that the latent goals of the organisation are more influential than those openly stated. Taken for granted latent goals may well be built into the fabric of the organisation.

When organisations present choices to their members, they may present either the loss or the gain as the dominant element according to the kind of institution. Some institutional types create problems that can best be solved by expansion (Douglas and Wildavsky, 1983: 89). So for example, in terms of obstetric practice in high-technology hospitals, problems of childbirth can only be dealt with through the expansion of instrumental and surgical intervention. The overwhelming advantages of expansion of obstetric services in risk management of maternity cases may be so dominant in everyone's minds that the gains would come to the fore in any presentation of a choice about alternative approaches, and the chances of losses, that is to the woman, would recede. On the other hand, people who have general confidence in the counteractive and anticipatory powers of their institutions may be disposed to estimate probabilities of loss differently from those people who mistrust their institutions. These three factors, the editing out of losses, the confidence in assessment procedures, and the feeling for future time, affect both estimated probabilities and magnitudes.

Cultural analysis does not ask about people's private beliefs. It asks what theories about the world emerge as guiding principles in a particular form of society. To apply this kind of analysis, Douglas and Wildavsky assume that a social form is always precarious because members of civil society try to alter it. Consequently there is always a debate about culture, about beliefs and values. If a social system remains stable over a period of time, twenty or thirty years, it is because the guardians of the present constitution were able to wrest control and gain public agreement to the supporting beliefs and values.

Western social thought, according to Douglas and Wildavsky (1983), habitually reverts to a typology of two, bureaucracy contrasted with the market. The organisational limits of these types are known, as is their style of decision-making, hidden assumptions and manifest priorities. An individual who spends her life exclusively in one or another such social environment internalises its values and bears its marks on her personality. It also follows that she will adopt the organisation's distinctive attitudes toward risks.

Bureaucratic behaviour is included under the more encompassing heading of hierarchy for the purposes of this analysis. Hierarchies include churches, industrial corporations, hospitals, and political hierarchies. They also include some forms of family and community organisations. Contrasted with hierarchies, Douglas and Wildavsky use individualism for the behaviour that includes the strategies of market orientation and sustained private self-interest. Each type creates a social environment in which distinctive strategies have to be adopted if both the individual member and the form of organisation are to survive.

The obstetric hierarchy has successfully endured over time and spread its area of control. In so doing it has managed to suppress internal and external rivalries so that influential individuals have been unable to disrupt its progress. Its success depends on not allowing one member's personal glory to be distinguished from the collective honour. Likewise no one member can be forced to take the blame provided they stay within the confines of the rules. Collective responsibility is undertaken by making roles anonymous. Decision-making should ideally be so collectivised that no one is seen to decide. If all operate on fixed instructions, everyone executes and no one decides policies (see Mannheim, 1960).

According to Frosch (1999) American specialists act as a cornerstone of international science, technology and health communities; 'communities that share a common culture across national boundaries and are thus themselves a force in the conduct of foreign policy' (ibid.: 16). Frosch provides some interesting statistics in the area of scientific and technical publications, for example, in 1981 The United States of America published 132,278, eight of which were jointly published with people from another country. By 1995 this figure had risen to 142,792 with only 19 internationally co-authored. By contrast, the United Kingdom published 30,794 in 1981 with only a small rise by 1995 (32,980). Of the latter only 29 were internationally co-authored. The former USSR, Germany and Japan published respectively 21,749, 30,634 and 39,498 (Frosch, ibid.).

North America, as the richest country, is well able to dispose some of its income on research, and is thus in a position to drive scientific, technical, health and childbirth ideology in whatever direction it chooses. The total number of articles published by authors in America, Europe, the former USSR and Canada taken together, amount to a 345,265 articles. In contrast, Asia (including Japan, China and India) only published 53,549 articles in 1995 and whilst not being insignificant may represent a much lesser degree of influence.

The struggle for a place in the global village

Within traditional cultures, the practices and beliefs surrounding pregnancy, childbirth, and early childhood development are passed on from one generation to another. When societies are more or less isolated from one another and outside influences are limited, what one generation passes on is similar to the way the next generation conducts their lives and actions, for example, in childbirth, and there is a relative stability of values, practices, and beliefs.

Traditional midwives are trained by their elders to facilitate the birth process, and to ensure the wellbeing of both the mother and the infant. They also provide the new mother and family with support during the infant's early life. There is a sense of continuity across time.

In many of the stories shared by women in Africa and Malaysia and even among women and midwives in Britain, I sensed a yearning for the world left behind (Laslett, 1999), a world that represented certainty, of knowing absolutely what the world was about. Instead, they viewed the world as being uncertain, strange. Many of the research participants expressed a feeling of being a 'stranger in a familiar place', of being alienated from their past, their culture, beliefs and understandings of the world around them. One respondent explained that she felt disorientated, confused, and being constantly anxious as a practitioner (Jo, Focus Group). The midwives in the focus group questioned the effect on their practice, 'I wonder whether this uncertainty makes our practice more dangerous rather than less' (Caroline, 1997). This feeling of uncertainty was evident in all the case study countries.

While some cultures have remained relatively isolated and intact, there are other cultures, which have been more vulnerable to change. This vulnerability is the result of increased exposure to other ideas, sometimes through formal education, and increasingly through mass media. For some societies the introduction of different ideas has resulted in a relatively easy incorporation of the new, with maintenance of the traditional. For others, the juxtaposition of the traditional and the new, along with economic changes which have threatened people's survival, has left cultures disorganised and people at a loss in terms of their values and beliefs. In the jargon of present-day psychology, these cultures could be classified as 'dysfunctional'. They are no longer able perhaps to provide the next generation with the grounding, stability, and vision that was found within traditional belief systems.

In the struggle for identity and in the desire to be 'modern', some have completely cast off their traditions, or think they have. Yet the modern does not always work for them. As a result, people are seeking to identify and recapture traditional values. There is an increasing awareness that much of what existed within traditional cultures was positive and supportive of growth and development, for the individual and for the society. Likewise there were practices that today we recognise as harmful to a person's health and wellbeing. It is this search to define and understand the traditional in relation to what is known today that is the basis of current research and programmes in many parts of the world.

Childbirth practices are embedded in a culture and determine, to a large extent, the behaviours and expectations surrounding a child's birth and infancy. While childbirth practices may be different across cultures, there are basic needs that all women have and predictable patterns of progression during labour that are universal. From the stories shared with me, it became very apparent that what women in childbirth claim to be important is a supportive and nurturing environment quite apart from adequate nutrition, health, and care following birth. Lack of support may have a significant effect on later health (see Oakley, 1992). Not only are there consequences for the woman's physical wellbeing; in addition, these variables interact with and have an impact on the woman's social and emotional wellbeing. While these factors are influenced by the economic and political context within which the woman lives, they are mediated through childbirth practices and beliefs.

In African, Malaysian, American and British societies the family, however defined, is the primary unit given responsibility for raising children. Within the cultures in this research, the community also had a clear role to play, whether to support women during childbirth as in Africa and Malaysia or to provide birthing systems. In pursuit of this task the family and community implement specific childbirth practices which they see as:

• ensuring the survival and health of the child; and
• ensuring the survival of the social group by assuring that women assimilate, embody and transmit appropriate social and cultural values through the process of childbirth.

To meet their goals, women in the case study countries adopted a set of practices, based on beliefs and values, from those made available to them through their culture. While women relied heavily on childbirth beliefs, which were a part of the culture, as the basis for their birth, there was considerable individual variation in practice, depending on the cultural group (Douglas and Wildavsky, 1983) to which the woman ascribed. The psychological characteristics of the woman, her previous experiences, and the conditions under which she was experiencing birth were all important factors in determining the outcome of birth. The role of other members of the society in childbirth differed depending on the specific cultural group, with community members playing a significant role in some settings and a more distant role in others.

It is not possible to define childbirth practices simply in relation to the ways in which the family and community function. The broader context that surrounds the family and community must also be taken into account. In societies with limited exposure to outside influences, the context is relatively constant, and as a result, childbirth practices remain more or less the same across generations. In societies in a state of rapid flux, such as Malaysia, there are dramatic changes from one generation to the next in the context within which childbirth occurs. In countries such as Ghana and Malawi, rapid flux and resultant changes happen more significantly in urban than in rural areas. Hospital births are much more common in urban centres, for example, while the majority of births still occur where the largest population resides, in the villages, attended by traditional midwives. These lead to differences in the type of care that is provided to women. From data collected during fieldwork,

I would conclude that the main areas where the context impacts upon childbirth practices and beliefs are as follows.

The context of the global village

Understanding the context helps provide an understanding both of the ways in which childbirth practices have developed and the ways in which they are evolving. The context is composed of many things and includes:

- the physical environment – the climate, geography of the area that determines the need for shelter from the heat or cold, and the relative ease of raising food crops to sustain the family; mobility. This is important for all the case study countries but for developing countries, poverty exacerbates any problems that might arise in the physical environment;
- the socio-political climate that determines whether women have security or a life dominated by fear; women's political voice; autonomy and power;
- the economic climate that determines women's abilities to survive and thrive; poverty and wealth; spending power;
- the philosophical and religious systems that provide a base for the values and beliefs of the society;
- the past, which is presented to the women through legends, myths, proverbs, riddles and songs that justify the existing social order and reinforce customs;
- the family and community who act as models of expected behaviour;
- the village, which presents a variety of situations calling for prescribed behaviour;
- the city that determines a different more hectic pace of life;
- technology and scientific advances;
- access to medical facilities; transportation and distance;
- women's control over their own bodies; freedom of choice;
- modern concepts of time.

The configuration of these dimensions determines the kinds of supports (or detractors) present as women give birth. One way to analyse possible configurations is along a continuum. In an analysis of childbirth practices in Africa, Malaysia, America and Britain, childbirth practices can be represented along a continuum related to degree of modernisation. At one end of the continuum are traditional cultures. These are defined as cultures within which childbirth practices and beliefs are based on inherited and orally transmitted knowledge. The context is more or less stable and there are adequate resources to support the traditional way of life. Such traditional cultures are more characteristic of rural than urban areas.

Negussie (1990) suggested that those migrating from rural to urban areas and/or living in marginal communities could be characterised as in transition, as in Malaysia. For these societies there is a shift away from traditional practices, especially in urban centres, as they are exposed to new ideas and/or there are changes in the environment, which threaten their survival, forcing them to make changes. Within societies that are in transition, childbirth practices and beliefs include a mix of the traditional and modern, and the mix is different depending on what is required of women.

The other end of the continuum can be defined as modern. Cultures located at this point on the continuum have access to and are using non-traditional health care and education in place of traditional systems. Negussie found that those living in peri-urban and urban areas, for example in Africa, or Malaysia, are most likely to be placed at this point on the continuum. I would argue that the continuum goes beyond the modern and into advanced modernity where post-industrial nations such as Britain and America have moved into an advanced technological era that some would describe as postmodern (Harvey, 1989; Leitch, 1996; Lyotard, 1984). This way of defining contexts is elaborated on below.

Traditional reliance on inherited and orally transmitted knowledge

In traditional society women in childbirth use imagery in many ways both to protect themselves and prepare themselves for giving birth. What a woman does, what she eats and the rituals that she undertakes are all opportunities for symbolically influencing herself and her unborn child. In the West we have forgotten the language of images, preferring instead to concentrate on analytical and explanatory modes of thought and communication. These are very necessary, of course, but are inadequate for communicating with ourselves and for viewing our situations and ourselves holistically. Many of the studies of childbirth beliefs and practices in Africa and Malaysia conducted last century captured the childbirth practices found within traditional societies (see Priya, 1992). Priya believes that we should learn from women in traditional societies and find ways of using images to engage with that part of our primal selves. Images can be used to change bodily processes in her view and we too should use these to help women give birth. Clearing doorways and untying knots are images used by women in childbirth in Malaysia and Africa but Priya urges Western women and those following the Western path to childbirth to find their own images derived from their experience of life in Western (modern) society.

While attending women in England, I frequently used the image of an opening flower to describe the process of cervical dilatation. I encouraged women to imagine this as they thought about their impending birth and 'see' their baby being easily delivered. On many occasions this appeared to work. The women tended to become more relaxed, their breathing changed and their labour progressed at an even pace. The images have to be useful and meaningful to the woman who uses them, however, and I encouraged women to create their own images and share these with their birth partner. Individual preparations of this nature, as Priya (1992: 130) asserts, cannot on their own foster a radical shift in childbirth practices in Britain, America or elsewhere where the Western model has been adopted. While childbirth continues to occur in hospitals where the ethos and physical focus are different and where power rests with the medical fraternity rather than the woman giving birth, then real change may be impossible.

In some countries there are pockets where these cultures continue to exist, but these are few and far between. In most countries, traditional childbirth practices, both positive and negative, are changing as women are exposed to other beliefs and practices. Where traditional practices have been interrupted the society may be classified as in transition. The effect of such a transition is manifested in the following areas.

1. CULTURAL SHIFTS IN A SOCIETY THAT RELIED PRIMARILY ON TRADITIONAL WISDOM AND NOW BEGINS TO ADOPT ALTERNATIVE BELIEFS AND PRACTICES

If the goals set by the 'modern society' are different from those of the indigenous society, the individual will usually follow the former. The result is often the disintegration of the earlier set of traditional goals and values. For Akinware and Ojomo (1993: 40) Nigerian society and culture is one undergoing such disintegration. The generally set goals seem to be Western, materialistic and individualistic. In the rural areas though, traditional values still seem to exist but these too are shaken by the principles of democratisation and modernisation, the vehicle of which is Western education.

Ghanaian, Malawian and Malaysian cultures can be characterised as in a time of transition as a result of the changes impacting on everyday life. These changes indirectly affect childbirth beliefs and practices and the growth and development of children. Women and their communities are in transition as a result of the following changes.

2. CHANGES IN THE TRADITIONAL FUNCTIONS OF THE FAMILY IN RESPONSE TO INVOLVEMENT WITH GLOBAL ORGANISATIONS, ECONOMY, POLITICS AND CULTURE

One particularly important support to women has been the community and the extended family system. In the past, close family ties provided a built-in measure of economic, emotional, and social security to women and families, but this traditional support for women has been disrupted as families move from rural to urban areas. Families migrate in search of work, and individual family members leave the village in search of educational and economic opportunities. Many of the previous roles of the community are being taken on by the wider society resulting in fragmentation, reduction in support systems and instability.

3. CHANGES IN THE STRUCTURE OF THE FAMILY

The size of families in the case study countries is declining. In Ghana, Malawi and Malaysia this is due partly to the fact that people are having fewer children, but more significantly the decline in family size is due to a move from multi-generational family groupings to the nuclear family. In Britain and America, increasing numbers of women are remaining childless and some women claim that they no longer think it necessary for them to have children to feel complete.

Women and girls have become the focus of international attention. Child rearing practices, which relied on the older girl child caring for younger children in the family, are being challenged. Girls who have traditionally been responsible for the care of younger siblings are attending school at an increased rate and being encouraged to complete their education. Consequently they are no longer available to care for younger siblings. Therefore women are losing a further source of support in the home.

4. CHANGES IN THE NATURE OF WOMEN'S WORK

Women all over the world have always played multiple roles that compete for their time and physical and emotional resources. Regardless of the context within which children are raised, care of children, particularly young children, is still the woman's responsibility. In addition, the woman is responsible for household management and operations, and economic/productive activity. New economic pressures on and possibilities presented to women mean that increasingly they work outside the home, often for long hours and following timetables that limit their availability and thus the time they can devote to family life.

In rural areas women often work in the fields. While in many cultures women have historically constituted a majority of the agricultural work force, in other settings the out-migration of men who are seeking employment has increased women's agricultural role. In addition, in some agricultural settings, plantation economies and cash crop production have meant that women are increasingly being exposed to the demands of rigid time and work schedules similar to those common in urban environments. In both urban and rural environments there is an increase in the number of woman-headed households. This inevitably has an impact on the woman's workload.

5. CHANGES IN MIGRATION PATTERNS

Until recently, men were the most likely to migrate in search of paid employment. In recent years, however, with the creation of free market zones, increasing numbers of women are migrating to obtain work. Women interviewed who had migrated to urban centres in Ghana, Malawi and Malaysia expressed nostalgia for the security of their old way of life and community, for within traditional societies, the norms, beliefs, and practices were relatively stable. Expectations in terms of childbirth behaviour were clear. For women in transition childbirth and child rearing practices are not clear. These women may lack the skills to live in the state of flux represented by transitional cultures. In this situation women may have a sense of powerlessness and be less self-confident in terms of their body skills. This can lead to childbirth practices that are inconsistent and/or overly restrictive. For those women who have been living in urban areas for a generation or two, they may well have incorporated more 'modern' childbirth beliefs and practices.

Migration and the distance between family members present major challenges to the maintenance of traditional practices despite the indication that some grandmothers are able to travel to the city to care for their daughters following delivery. To quote one grandmother:

> I travelled to the United States of America for the birth of my granddaughter. We were able to conduct the rites as we do here. My daughter was able to have a complete rest and I taught her the traditional ways.
> (Chan, 1994, Malaysia)

Moreover, female employment in the formal sector is directly pertinent to grandmothers who work and are unable to take time from their jobs to provide the traditional care for their daughters or daughters-in-law.

Modernity: when non-traditional health, education and social supports are available and relied upon more than the traditional

Technology has made a wide variety of supports available to families that are not available within traditional cultures. While there are advantages and disadvantages to every piece of technology that has been introduced, the availability of these technologies has radically changed people's lives. For example, bottle-feeding has made it easier for women to enter the labour market. But the introduction of bottle-feeding and the decrease in breastfeeding has resulted in high infant mortality and morbidity rates due to improper use of bottles and infant formula in some developing countries.

Modern women are defined by their openness to new experiences, including family planning and birth control. Their assertion of increasing independence from traditional authority figures and belief in the efficacy of science and technology leads to an abandonment of passivity and fatalism. Modern women are ambitious for their children to achieve higher educational and occupational goals as was identified in the analysis of six women's roles in the Malaysian case study.

It is interesting to note that the traditional and modern Malaysian families were only one generation apart. The parents of the more modern women who were included in the study were non-literate farmers from the traditional village in the study. Thus, while in some instances there are several generations between the traditional societies and the modern, this movement has generally occurred within only one generation.

The negative aspects of globalisation noted in the case study countries included the following.

- A dehumanisation of the social environment (with increased use of the bottle rather than the breast; babies left with other carers rather than carried on their mothers' backs; and a reliance on mass media rather than human interaction for entertainment). For women in childbirth, the dehumanisation process was reflected in the impersonal treatment of women, standardised care, routinisation of practices which were claimed to be individual but were in fact standardised to a set formula for care in childbirth. Women were frequently separated from their social support networks in hospital settings in Africa and Malaysia, sometimes being left unattended in corridors or in the middle of large labour rooms to labour in public without attendants to nurture them. (When visiting a major city hospital in Ghana, however, I found a group of pregnant women sitting under a large shady tree, cooking, washing clothes and generally camping out. When asked, my guide explained that they were squatting there waiting to go into labour so that their babies could be born in hospital. This was seen as high status.)

- The disintegration of family and community units and of commitment to each other. Smaller units of ownership and residence lead to less sharing and more individualism. There was an expression of a distinct loss of community among participants in the study. In Ghana, however, elements of this community feeling still existed and were manifested in ordinary people willing to share whatever they had with friends and strangers alike.

- Decrease in traditional education mirrors the increase in modern education. Consequently traditional knowledge is being reduced (closing of the mind) not without consequences for women in childbirth. The traditional methods of child spacing served their purpose so long as taboos, rules and traditions were observed. With the introduction of instrumentalism in fertility control have come pressures that have reduced the respect for and contribution of these traditional practices, especially in urban areas. The increase in modern education and decrease in traditional education has also played its part. Many people do not know about traditional methods of fertility control and the lack of sex education in schools has resulted in an increase in the numbers of unwanted pregnancies, pregnancies outside marriage and pregnancies and births that are too close, especially in urban settings.

In sum, in Ghanaian, Malawian and Malaysian cultures great importance is placed on having children. Thus it is not surprising that there are numerous beliefs and rituals that support the birth and raising of a healthy child.

This study has revealed that traditional childbirth practices in different parts of the world continue, although the forces of modernisation have influenced them. For example, pregnancy is no longer as sensitive a subject as it was. The reason for this is that there is considerable modern information available and being provided to women. When they receive this information they are encouraged to talk about their own situation. Pregnant women, for example, are now eating foods which they are advised will benefit the unborn child, although traditionally these foods were taboo.

Traditional practices related to the birth of the child are still persistent, with traditional midwives and close relatives playing a crucial role in helping to deliver the child. However, increasingly children are being born in health facilities and the traditional practices are not being followed. Also, the 'confinement' period is breaking down for those who deliver their children in the hospital or birthing clinic. This is due to short hospital stays and being exposed to the public on discharge from the maternity hospital.

The rites and observances emphasise equal care and attention for the mother and child during the puerperium, instead of concentration on the child to the neglect of the mother, as in the American health care system. A reduction in postnatal services is also creeping into the British maternity care services partly as a result of budgetary constraints. Puerperal rites and practices promote cross-generational maternal health. They provide a unique opportunity for the young, inexperienced mother to learn about baby care, family and home management in their home. This promotes child and family health both directly and indirectly. These rites provide older women with a new and highly valued role within the family and society, contributing greatly to their self-esteem, reputation, and general wellbeing. During the puerperal period the grandmother is the figure of authority within the family. This teaches children to cherish, respect and trust older women. In this way, these rites create a bond between the woman's nuptial and natal families, and thus enhance family life and social integration. On the societal level, these rites clearly underscore the crucial importance of the neonatal period for the survival of human beings and society as has been shown by demographic and medical research. Under the conditions of modernity the prospects for the survival of these birth rites is in the balance. There are three obstacles in modern African and Malaysian society to obtaining support for the mother and the observance of rites of passage in the postnatal period, namely female employment in the formal sector, urbanisation, and migration out of the villages.

In sum, there are instances where more 'modern' practices are replacing traditional practices. In some instances the replacements are of benefit to the mother and child, as in the situation where women have more information about conception, pregnancy, and the birth process, and they are using this information to assure the birth of a health baby and to take care of themselves physically. However, there are a number of instances where more 'modern' practices have supplanted the traditional and this has had a negative impact on the child and/or the mother. This is true in the case of child spacing and the introduction of bottle-feeding.

Discussion

It is against the background of individualisation as a process that calls for increased self-responsibility and self-reflexivity that dominant tendencies in the theory and practice of obstetrics are to be understood. From this perspective it is also understandable that obstetrics concentrates upon the individual survival of women in the turmoil of risks and chances involved in the lifestyles that belong to the risk society. And it is only a logical development, in accordance with processes of individualisation, that childbirth has applied itself to a diversification and individualisation. Depending on the specific circumstances and practical needs of the women, the provision of maternity care in the Western world is offered in new 'tailor-made' forms and concepts, like epidural birth; instrumental birth; caesarean section births – 'to keep the honeymoon passage fresh' as one billboard proclaims in the USA; standardised hospital birth; birth centres; home birth and home-like births in hospital; domino delivery; Lamaze birth; active childbirth; water birth and so on. In a way this seems a necessary and pertinent response to the challenges of the risk society. So one might rightly claim that these new practices and concepts in maternity care are significant institutional adjustments to the highly individualised childbirth needs of today's society. But at the same time these practices and concepts confirm and reinforce the ongoing processes of individualisation. For that reason, obstetric practice and midwifery might also be considered as a medium that intensifies the characteristic experiences of self-responsibility in the risk society.

The unique experiences of women in rural areas of Africa, Malaysia and among the Amish in America show a different picture. Traditional midwives have a long-established knowledge of the women and families in their localities. They are able to 'speak their lineage' in a way that midwives in urban settings are unable to do. Mary, the Amish midwife in Pennsylvania, for example, had lived and worked in her community all her life. She knew every person, their health and social histories, their problems and their joys. Every birth was recorded by the women she had delivered on a quilt on which the names of the babies and parents and dates of birth were embroidered on squares in a colourful history of childbirth. Mary was able to tell the stories of every birth and the history of the families from looking at the quilt.

Florence, a traditional midwife in Malawi was able to name every person in her village and recount their histories. She not only knew that a labouring mother had had more than the usual amount of blood loss following her last delivery but also that the woman's own mother and grandmother had the same experience. Florence was prepared for the possible repeat of such an event, 'The women in that family always bleed too much – so I give them herbal medicine to prevent it' (Florence, 1991, Malawi). The herbal remedy used was a secret but the nurse-midwife revealed that she knew that it was a mixture of papaya leaves and other herbs that helps the uterus to contract and so hinders bleeding.

The majority of the population in African countries and to a significant extent in Malaysia still reside in rural areas. On the whole, foreign health researchers comfortably place themselves away from the common people's reach. Increasingly, indigenous people who are obtaining their scientific education in health, become involved in different policy planning meetings, dialogue with different scientific and literate communities and implement finely-tuned strategies and technologies that are all aimed towards the development of health practitioners of the country. In the process, however, they often ignore women's knowledge and their own aspirations, culture, tradition, age-old knowledge and beliefs. The result has been short-term progress in reduction of maternal and neonatal mortality and fertility rates but the gains have not been sustained.

An African focus group of senior nurse-midwives made the point that:

> Western researchers believe that their approach is purely scientific. They tend to disregard women's knowledge as non-specific and based on traditional faiths that have no significant importance in the age of modern-day scientific advancement.
>
> (Ghana, 1991)

Sometimes, as a convention and as warranted by different development programmes, researchers engage in learning a practitioner's local knowledge but they may fail to completely realise its meaning and relevance to such development efforts as some may stay isolated from the local environment and the people by either not living in the community or being mentally and emotionally distant from it, perhaps to maintain a sense of objectivity. On the other hand, African researchers with a background in modern Western style education readily become influenced by Western culture and begin craving for the urban lifestyle that consciously or unconsciously places them at odds with the heritage, culture and traditions of rural people. Those researchers who become absorbed with their own short-term goals and preferences may become blind to the world beyond. They may fail to take account of the fact that local practitioners, with their roots embedded in that particular locality, could provide the information needed for exploration by the outsider, the one-time researcher. This may well be, in fact, a by-product of a particular feature of modernity – specialisation.

Moghaddam (1997: 9) reminds us that we place considerable faith in experts – one of the products of increasing specialisation. Out of a lack of confidence, a lack of skill, respect for science, fear of authority, or simply being too lazy to think for ourselves, we rely on experts rather than on our own insights. We now seem to need experts to tell us, for example, that pollution is destroying the ecological balance on earth; that infants are healthier when they are loved; that the family does have an important social role in the development of children and that the health and education systems are in trouble. What may be obvious to us only achieves the status of 'truth' when endorsed by experts. It is interesting to consider this statement in view of the almost manic demand for 'evidence-based practice' in health care globally. Socialisation processes in modern societies are such that when faced with even the slightest personal or societal issue, people often look to experts for answers. Modern cultural habits, which are particularly apparent in the United Kingdom and the United States, tend to transform every moral crisis into a technical problem for which there should be an expert solution.

For the rich, the experts are available through private consultations, for which they are charged vast fees. But experts have also made themselves available to the masses, through the mass media and through thousands of 'self-help' publications. The Internet now places thousands of 'experts' all over the world at the fingertips of anyone who has access. Without these information sources, it seems, it would be impossible for us to do anything well, from building cabinets to having children. But the credibility of experts has not entirely escaped questioning, a fact made apparent by the common wisdom in many different cultures 'that a person may know a great deal in a narrow field but is, in fact, an idiot'.

Expertise and 'power to the people'

The general mistrust of the 'idiot expert' is often coupled with a call for the 'empowerment' of the general public, to put lay-people on a more equal footing with experts. Based on the dictum, 'Knowledge is power', this movement involves efforts to provide the public with more medical, legal and other types of information that have traditionally been monopolised by professionals. Presumably, by more fully informing the public about various important issues, we help to transfer power from experts to lay-people. Such empowerment strategies gained momentum in the 1960s and have sub-sequently become particularly strong in the areas of environmental protec-tion and animal rights, although the issue of power relations between experts and the public is by no means the exclusive concern of modern societies.

In America and Britain, what has become increasingly apparent is that women, particularly middle-class women, are informing themselves about childbirth, their rights and choices, to a much higher degree than those encountered five years ago. With the advent of the Internet, women have comparatively easy access to a much broader range of information from all over the world. It is interesting, however, that the Americans dominate the Internet with much less information coming from other countries. This might be viewed yet again as a way in which American ideology and culture is transmitted globally. It is important to note that the Internet, however, gives easier access to a platform for alternative ideologies to be expressed than other media forms, since it is not censored and controlled by the dominant medical organisations and publications. Thus, one could argue, women are exposed to ideas and values that would have otherwise been screened and hidden from them.

In terms of 'knowledge as power', however, I would argue that it is only authenticated, authoritative knowledge held by people in power positions that is powerful (see Jordan, 1993; Davis-Floyd, 1997). Traditional midwives' knowledge is not power – midwifery knowledge is not power – women's knowledge is not power, because their knowledge has little status within the dominant scientific system and so they are not recognised as authentic creators or controllers of knowledge.

Conclusion

In the environment of modern obstetrical care the support and confidence that women need to give birth successfully is often destroyed or diminished. They find it harder to give birth without medical intervention. The advent of the globalisation of modernity in the wake of different colonial experiences has brought with it an orientation held by medical men and midwives of the superiority of Western health delivery systems.

In Africa and Malaysia, many of the Western educated practitioners I came across regarded indigenous knowledge as native tales, proverbs, and sayings of some rural illiterates that were mostly devoid of any scien-tific foundation or signification. Thus, in those countries well planned scien-tifically conceived programmes, for example, TBA training, ended up as failures since those programmes were planned in city-based offices by high-technology personnel who failed to listen to rural people.

In the wake of the economic downturn experienced in Malaysia and Africa, however, there has been a turn-around in the utilisation of indigenous knowledge and technologies. There is a wealth of indigenous knowledge held by traditional midwives and healers that could be blended with modern scientific evidence to produce technologies that are relevant, affordable and sustainable in an African setting.

It is clear from discussions with local people that the influence of Western science and more significantly the value placed on measurements, is increasingly changing the ways of thinking about childbirth in both the developed and developing countries under study.

Chapter 9

Cultural implications for midwifery education and practice

It is increasingly important that the midwifery curriculum is grounded within an understanding of the social and economic history of our times and the salience of markets, privatisation and globalisation. Formal education does not function in a vacuum and a curriculum is always performed in a physical, social and cultural context that is subject to both internal and external forces as described in the preceding chapters. Curriculum is thus contextually shaped and globally influenced.

Midwifery education is defined as the study of childbirth and midwifery issues aimed at developing the theoretical, conceptual and practical framework of, and for, the education of practitioners of midwifery. In the past few years the shift towards delivering the midwifery curriculum in or affiliated to universities is part of a general shift in the changing role of higher education worldwide. There are eight key concerns, as follows, that impact upon and shape the nature of midwifery education and the curriculum to varying degrees in all five case study countries, namely Ghana, Malawi, Malaysia America and England.

Global interconnectedness: local reframing

- Women's issues; status – degree of power and authority; choice; control, needs and wants; wealth/poverty; health.
- The communication revolution; mass media; World Wide Web and Internet; availability and easy access to information for self-diagnosis.
- Economics and marketplace, global corporations, competition; mobility of work force; access to money and resources.
- The knowledge explosion; scientific and technological developments; emphasis on research and evidence-based practice; specialisation.
- Ecological imperatives; planetary resources and hazards; pollution; impact on health and women in childbirth.
- Increasing pluralism; shift from community-based focus to individual focus.

- Search for meaning, personal achievements; cultural alignment to particular cultural types.
- Societal changes, towards increasing litigation; desire for the exotic; desire for modernity; risk society.

These factors have been examined in the preceding chapters. Now we move on to the following questions. What are the cultural implications for midwifery education? What does this mean for the development of educational programmes for midwives globally?

The cultural implications of modernity for the education and training of midwifery practitioners

Modernity and education have developed simultaneously, acting on and reacting to each other. The technological development that ushered in the modern age created the demand for high levels of education. Education, in turn, has trained people not only to use technology but also to go on and develop new and higher forms. Thus, modernity's technical foundation both creates and depends on advanced systems of education, which in turn, create and depend on technology.

As societies develop and change under the impact of globalisation and new knowledge becomes available, the content of education likewise changes. In the modern world the greatest advantage a nation or individual can possess is access to and participation in symbolic-analytic services. Symbolic-analytic services are problem-solving, problem-identifying, and strategic brokering activities in which symbols – data, words, and visual representations – are manipulated. As Reich explained, symbolic analysts:

> simplify reality into abstract images that can be rearranged, juggled, experimented with, communicated to other specialists, and then, eventually transformed back into reality. The manipulations are done with analytic tools, sharpened by experience. The tools may be mathematical, algorithms, legal arguments, financial gimmicks, scientific principles, psychological insights about how to persuade or amuse, systems of induction or deduction, or any other set of techniques for doing conceptual puzzles.
>
> (Reich, 1991: 178)

This type of work is performed in a variety of occupations in science, engineering, law, public relations, management, energy, architecture, agriculture, marketing, the media, higher education and elsewhere. Practitioners in these fields find ways of increasing efficiency, yielding greater resources, saving time, or creating something new altogether. While most countries, including America, tend to teach a prescribed standardised curriculum, Reich found that, although in mathematics and science American high school students often lag behind their counterparts in Japan, South Korea, Great Britain and Germany, the best students in America were better prepared for symbolic analysis than in any other country in the world.

Embryonic symbolic analysts learn to construct meanings for themselves; provide their own interpretations; organise information; and identify new solutions, problems, and choices. This entails, as stated by Reich (1991: 229), refining four basic skills:

- abstraction;
- system thinking;
- experimentation;
- collaboration.

Abstraction is the ability to take disorganised information, integrate and assimilate it, and shape it into a workable and perhaps original pattern. Students are not given pre-digested information nor are they required to commit it to memory in order to become adept at abstraction; rather they learn to interpret data and give meaning to it themselves. To promote this process the curriculum needs to be fluid and interactive.

> Instead of emphasising the transmission of information, the focus is on judgement and interpretation. The student is taught to get behind the data – to ask why certain facts have been selected, why they are assumed to be important, how they were deduced, and how they might be contradicted. The student learns to examine reality from many angles, in different lights, and thus to visualise new possibilities and choices. The symbolic-analytic mind is trained to be sceptical, curious, and creative.
>
> (Reich, 1991: 230)

Another characteristic of symbolic analysis is system thinking. This is an extension of abstraction in that it involves the ability to visualise how the various components of an object, issue, or problem are linked together. Thus the symbolic analyst tries to discern 'larger causes, consequences, and relationships' (Reich, ibid.: 231). In system thinking, students are taught not to immediately solve problems that are presented to them, but to examine why the problem arises and how it is connected to other problems. Solutions can therefore be more effectively determined, as they are based on a consideration of a broad range of possible variables, influences and outcomes.

System thinking and abstraction are learned through experimentation; students test and explore various possibilities or outcomes, noting similarities and differences, in seeking the best possibility or outcome for a particular situation. Finally Reich notes a capacity for collaboration, or the ability to communicate abstract concepts, to negotiate needs, to seek and accept criticism from peers, and to work as part of a group. In this model learning does not cease on graduation, but continues on the job since much of the work symbolic analysts engage in is oriented toward creative problem solving and gaining new insights.

America does not have a monopoly on symbolic analysts; however, the direction of the most modern forms of education across the globe appears to be towards producing more symbolic analysts. Modernity rests on advanced educational systems, and the social change it produces is based on the production of new knowledge. Thus modernity and education are invariably linked; one builds on the other. In all societies education has become increasingly important. Advanced nations, in particular, have found that ever-larger proportions of their populations are employed in jobs that require well-educated workers.

In the past, such mechanistic interpretations of human behaviour, promoted by sensualism, associationism and behaviourism, have compartmentalised human activities, and consequently have led to the development of separate sciences, such as biology, psychology, and sociology. Implied in these approaches is the tendency to segregate parts and components analytically. Little attention was given – and little success was achieved – in putting the pieces together again. The main task of science can be seen to be to disintegrate Humpty Dumpty (Riegel, 1978: 15).

Modern midwifery theory and practice are rooted in the biological sciences and the enhanced understanding of these has had a major impact upon the organisation and delivery of midwifery and obstetric education and practice.

Midwifery education and practice: sociocultural determinants

Midwifery education and practice has, until latterly, been more or less confined within the boundaries of the national context. Granted there has been sharing across boundaries and the influence of the World Health Organization and the International Confederation of Midwives cannot be denied. But generally speaking, apart from the influence of midwifery consultants, under the auspices of such global agencies, on the developing world, there has been little interconnection between midwifery programmes of study. The formal, organised midwifery curriculum has generally been influenced by local and national considerations and by statutory requirements. In the West, under the influence of science and technology we have seen an increasing industrialisation of childbirth along with increased instrumentalism that has, in effect, created a distance between midwives and the women they attend. Figure 9.1 attempts to illustrate the potential and real effects of modernity and globalisation upon the knowledge and values underpinning the curriculum.

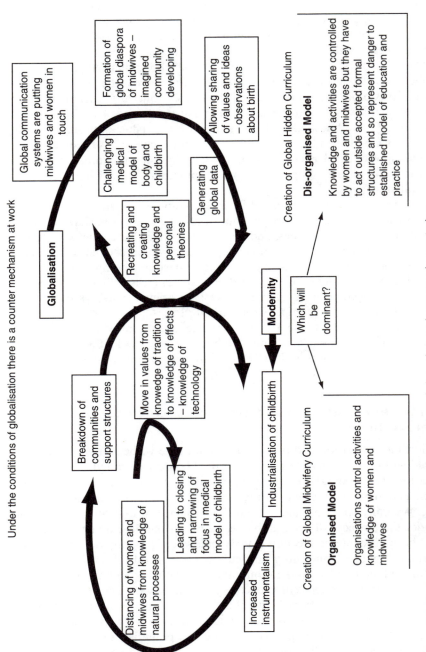

Figure 9.1 Modernity and globalisation: impact on knowledge, values underpinning the curriculum

One of the prime effects of this distancing has been to prevent midwives and women from developing and understanding the ways in which women's bodies work. Midwives working in the industrialised model of childbirth, especially in the context of hospital services, seldom have enough time to devote to a single woman throughout her pregnancy, labour and delivery to generate a personal theory of the interconnectedness between the woman's body and that of her unborn child. Industrialised childbirth moreover, replaces or excludes the valuable supportive social networks that play such an important role in childbirth in the villages in Africa, the kampongs in Malaysia and among the Amish community in America.

Most of the nascent midwife's knowledge comes instead from de-contextualised theory leading to a narrowing of focus and a closing of the mind which may be influenced by experiences of horizontal violence (see Leap, 1997; McCall, 1996). As midwives become increasingly removed from the community context of childbirth they lose the integrated knowledge of the unity of mind and body. They gain more technical knowledge but lose social knowledge. The result is a closing of the mind – if it is not directly relevant to the physical work of childbirth then it is irrelevant. We are experiencing a shift in values from knowledge of tradition to knowledge of effects and knowledge of technology along with the breakdown in community and support structures. As the medical model of childbirth is transmitted globally, these effects will multiply as health institutions and hospitals gain increasing control over childbirth, women and midwives.

There is, however, a growing counter-current in that under the conditions of globalisation with its increased communication networking, midwives, or at least those who are able to access the global networks, are communicating directly with each other – by-passing official institutions and developing a knowledge-base that is not necessarily legitimated by authoritative agencies. Nonetheless, the mere act of writing down and sharing information about practice with other midwives and women around the world is, perhaps, beginning to formulate a legitimate body of knowledge that challenges the dominant medical model. Certainly, questions and challenges to the medical establishment are being put forward both by women and midwives, one only has to look at the midwifery web pages to appreciate the extent of this activity. In consequence, what we are beginning to see is a global hidden curriculum developing that is beyond the control of socialising agents, but generally, those midwives and women who wish to practice alternative approaches to childbirth in America and England, still have to do so outside the mainstream organisations.

Making midwives: traditional birth attendant training

Governments and development institutions view the training of TBAs as an aspect of health service delivery. Accordingly, they define birth assistance as 'medical', whether or not the people involved define the practices associated with birth in terms of health and sickness. In Ghana, Malawi and Malaysia women who perform a ritual service become defined, for the purposes of training, as midwives who perform medical services. A spectrum of birth-related concerns, spanning issues of ritual pollution, the vulnerability of pregnant women and infants to witchcraft, to issues of modesty and embarrassment are reorganised in the framework for training TBAs. Within local understanding, for instance, the main role of the woman who cuts the birth cord may be to carry away the ritual pollution associated with birth. For many Ghanaians and Malaysians ideas about witchcraft and pollution are as real as a placenta.

In effect, training programmes redefine the practices of the trainees. Birth is easier to speak about than African and Malaysian notions about spirits that cause illnesses, for instance. Everyone can agree, for example, whether or not the placenta has been delivered, while no such agreement is possible for the chasing away of ghosts. There is predictability to the known events of pregnancy and childbirth and concrete techniques for dealing with them. As a consequence, TBA and midwifery training programmes work with a presumed common and obvious concern with the management of pregnancy, labour and birth.

The development perspective, consequently, regards the traditional midwife's role only as a potentially medical one, in which the main purpose is to safeguard the health of mother and child. In general, all practices are treated as if they fit a common idealised role of 'midwife,' even though it is well known in international policy circles that not all 'birth attendants' fit the image of the midwife who cares for a woman throughout the pregnancy, birth, and postpartum period. Training programmes are nevertheless structured so as to re-create systematically the trainees in the image of the traditional midwife. Trained TBAs and midwives are fashioned as technicians and the varying social, emotional, protective, or polluting roles the trainees might actually be playing are subsumed under the role of managing birth itself.

The 'obviousness' of this common reality is deceptive. Different cultures understand, organise and manage birth in their own way (see Jordan 1993). Anthropologists insist that the social aspect of birth can never be separated from its physiological aspect, for the physical events of childbirth always take place within a shared understanding of 'the best way, the right way, indeed the only way to bring a child into the world' (Jordan, ibid.: 4).

TBA training, however, is based on the notion that the 'cultural' dimension of childbirth can be separated from the 'physiological' dimension. While careful not to interfere with beliefs and customs if they are deemed 'harmless,' they introduce a biomedical understanding of birth through the back door by focusing on a physiological realm separated from social considerations. Training programmes for midwives as a whole convey a biomedical ideology not simply through the theories of physiology and disease causation they teach but also through the insistence in the format of training themselves that the physiological be clearly separated from social, moral, and religious concerns. These are the very people who take responsibility for training TBAs. The medicalisation of birth attendants, tacitly enacted through training, requires trainees themselves to fragment their practices, distinguishing between the 'medical' and the 'social' aspects of what they do.

There are aspects of Ghanaian, Malawian and Malaysian women's practices that are left out or marginalised in training programmes, precisely because of the importance placed on techniques and physiology. Nowhere is there a space created for the emotional and social significance of birth. This accounts, I believe, for some of the astonishing omissions in discussions of 'local ideas and practices'. The many ways Ghanaians, for example, give special care to pregnant women, new mothers and babies' vanish in development accounts. How they show care can only be grasped within the framework through which they themselves perceive dangers and problems. An example from fieldwork is captured in the following description of a birth I attended in Ghana.

Dora's story

Crouched in the corner of the dark hut, the TBA sat and waited quietly. I sat in the opposite corner and watched, silently. The woman lay on her side, labouring without a sound. Outside we could hear the singsong voices of the women as they stirred the pot of porridge they had prepared for the labouring woman to keep her strength up. They were waiting for the birth and from time to time one or other of them would come into the hut to quietly give support. Through the touch of a hand, a stroke of her brow, giving a sip of water or porridge, they expressed their caring, their concern and their connectedness to the event. This sisterhood was an important part of the ritual of birth. It seemed to be significant in relaxing the woman and perhaps even reducing her pain. The men were not present – this was women's work. The TBA did not examine the woman or take measurements of her pulse or blood pressure every fifteen minutes, there was no external monitor beeping away in the background. The scene was startling in its quiet peacefulness – its lack of intrusion.

(Dora's birth experience, Ghana, 1991)

Cross-cultural research on childbirth has shown just how historically specific the notion of medically managed childbirth is (see Jordan, 1993). A medicalised construction of pregnancy and childbirth dictates that these states must be managed and monitored by specialists. In the United States and United Kingdom, in fact, women who give birth without professional management are regarded as negligent (Tsing, 1990). Furthermore, obstetricians tend to treat women in labour as unruly 'workers' who must be monitored in case they damage 'the product' (Martin, 1987). Emily Martin has shown that the time-management and efficiency approach that breaks the process of childbirth down into stages facilitates the comparison, evaluation, and control of women in labour. Tacitly, childbirth that is not supervised by a trained expert is considered suspect, both in the United Kingdom and the United States.

These deeply ingrained cultural assumptions are being transferred to developing countries in notions about how birth is best managed. The fact of expert management itself may be as important to this moralistic sense of what is 'best' as the actual techniques that might have positive effects on maternal and infant mortality. TBAs are looked to as the experts who can adopt the role of manager. Public health nurses can, in turn, supervise their practice on behalf of development institutions.

Finally, the structure of a training programme itself communicates certain messages to the trainees. For Ghanaian, Malawian and Malaysian women, training programmes are features of a wider world of 'development' and 'modernity.' They are but one aspect of a larger process in Ghana, Malawi and Malaysia by which being 'modern' becomes associated with a higher social status (see Pigg, 1992). When women attend training programmes they learn what 'modern' people are supposed to do and say. This knowledge is authoritative for these women not simply because the trainers present it as such but because training comes out of institutions that are creating an authority for 'developed' ideas overall. What is learned in training has more relevance in the context of status negotiation, where it matters socially that one appears 'developed,' than it does in the contexts in which births actually take place. Training programmes thus widen women's senses of the disparity between 'modern' practices and their (now devalued) local realities.

In considering how authoritative knowledge is displayed in interactions, we need to look beyond the rooms where birth takes place to the other sites where authority is produced and reproduced. Training is one such site, to which I turn next.

Knowledge production in development ideology

The irony here is that in the attempt to create programmes tailored to local conditions, a great deal of what local people think, believe and do is filtered out through the circulation of information about the 'local' in the apparatuses of development knowledge. The authoritative knowledge about childbirth communicated in training is linked to the production of authoritative knowledge about 'local ideas and practices'. It is therefore important to understand the process that produces the knowledge of 'traditional beliefs and practices' on which 'culturally appropriate' health development is based. The discursive regulation of what can be said in development begins in the regulation of what can be known.

The research techniques used to gather baseline information and evaluate programme effectiveness already screen what is considered relevant and irrelevant information. Questionnaires, surveys, and focus groups are designed with certain ideas about 'traditions' already in mind. In this process, a mobile, dislocated concept of tradition comes to be filled with the facts from Ghana, Malawi and Malaysia.

The authoritative knowledge about local practices that is presented in reports fundamentally alters these practices by inventing new terms in which they can make sense. Facts are selected and rearranged in a way that produces an image of 'local tradition' for development observers that not only distorts local practices out of recognition but also virtually ensures that local ideas are silenced and excluded from development. In the process of collecting, summarising, and analysing data some aspects of local reality pass easily from one stage of reformulation to another, attaining the status of information about local ideas and practices, while other aspects remain silent and invisible. One thing that occurs to me is how or whether the discourse of anthropology has informed ideas about traditional birth practices. Western anthropological models tend to focus on concerns such as prohibitions and rituals, that is the classic subject matter of anthropology, and not on other issues. Could it be that anthropology has influenced what is looked for in terms of local practices? For example, because Evans-Pritchard ([1937] 1972) talked about Azande witchcraft, everybody else looks for witchcraft, even if it is 'not there' or could more sensibly be described in another way.

The first question most development observers ask about a custom or a practice is 'Does this do harm?' This is of course an important question to ask. But being too quick to seize on 'harmful customs' blinds us to the wider context in which these practices occur. These are then readily translated into training programmes.

There is more than insensitivity or misuses of words at stake here. Translations circulate endlessly through what teachers ask students and what teachers hear students say. Training occurs, moreover, in contexts in which public health trainers, whose native language is not English, are taught using terms that are specific to development jargon (for example, TBA). These workers then use this terminology with villagers who consult them, turning abbreviations such as TBA into words. Even when specific indigenous words are retained, their meaning inevitably changes when interspersed in the English utterances of a foreign official, or institutionalised in the development office jargon of Ghanaian, Malawian and Malaysian staff. Such abbreviations are essentially reductionist in nature –for both the term and the practice are reduced to the base elements.

The issue is not one of correctness or authenticity in language use but of social relations, institutional procedures and power. Discourse has concrete consequences. Villagers find themselves having to interact with development institutions that have structured their programmes around static and distorted representations of 'tradition'. To obtain desired resources they have to construct themselves in the way development has 'imagined' traditional people to be. Development persuades local realities to conform to development categories, and only those aspects of local reality that can be successfully disguised in these categories can be incorporated in programmes and planning.

Paradoxically, development practices of knowledge production help to perpetuate the 'gap' between planning and local realities that so concerns development planners. This gap is the product of systematic techniques for framing and understanding 'local ideas and practices'. The language used in development work becomes entangled with actual institutional practices, and together they reiterate what Wood (1985) called the 'delinking' of people from their social context. This 'delinking' has an effect on several levels according to Pigg (1995). Noticeably, it facilitates bureaucratic administration by narrowing the vision of complex realities. Yet, at the same time, the resultant simplification that facilitates administrative plans generates problems of programme implementation in the field. When development programmes based on decontextualised, distorted notions of 'traditional ideas and practices' are set in motion in actual villages they face numerous practical problems. Important messages fail to be communicated effectively. Even programmes explicitly planned with 'traditional ideas and practices' and 'the local level' in mind fall far short of 'bridging the gap' in the way intended. The decontextualization resulting from the practices of translation detailed above detracts from the programme effectiveness even as it serves bureaucratic purposes. It is difficult for development institutions to really resolve these contradictions, for 'delinking' also serves a greater ideological purpose by positioning development itself as transcendent and authoritative.

This heightened focus on TBAs is a function of the distinction made in development discourse between its own role as a catalytic force coming from 'outside' and the inner world of closed traditional societies (Pigg, 1995). The picture of global social differences created by implication a role for mediators and cultural brokers. TBAs were imagined to fit perfectly in this interstitial space. They had similar concerns and interests, allegedly, as fellow health promoters, but were dissimilar to educated professional practitioners in that they were characterised as trusted cultural insiders who were able to carry development messages into the unseen heart of traditional societies. The shift towards treating traditional practitioners as a resource, was part of the cycle in development through which past mistakes became lessons that continually provided new and improved solutions. It therefore increased the appearance of progressive advancement on which development rests. Regardless of where people are located in the world, their experiences tend now to reflect the culmination of a shift in their consciousness and they almost all now view themselves in direct relation to an explicit image of modern life.

Under the collective rationality of the development model both policy and implementation, subsume 'local tradition'. Training programmes, while

aiming to enhance the expertise of local practitioners, require that participants understand that whole areas of their experience and knowledge are
irrelevant to the development context. Local practitioners are both portrayed
as, and made into, people whose knowledge has a limited, local importance.

Development programmes seldom work as imagined. The usual response
to the disjuncture between the assumptions behind development programmes
and the realities of local life has been to instigate more and better research
about local ideas and practices. Even when such information is provided,
however, it is rarely used effectively, as Justice's work (1984, 1986, 1994) on
development bureaucracies has shown. The persistent assumption is that
adjustments made to the development model would resolve its inherent
problems.

Pigg (1995) suggested that the development paradigm, with its prescribed
formulae for cultural beliefs and practices, should be abandoned. Instead,
other vocabularies for framing concerns about health and culture should
be developed. In rushing to provide better 'sociocultural information',
researchers and planners fail to question how the very definition of 'sociocultural' is constrained by development interests. The language used by
development agencies is produced by and reproduces a power asymmetry that
becomes more entrenched every time development visions turn into policies
and policies turn into actual programmes. It is past time to consider that
development discourse also produces distinctive problems, and in fact these
problems are necessary to development power and must be perpetually
recreated to sustain it.

Development mediates the circulation of differing medical modes, ensuring
that those deemed traditional remain local, limited, and context-specific
while modern medicine acquires a global and universal role. This is how
cosmopolitan obstetrics becomes, in Jordan's (1993: 199–214) words, a cosmopolitical obstetrics whose authority rests on a certain distribution of
power. At present in mainstream international health development other
modes of knowledge are recognised as 'different' and granted a limited
sphere of authority within the bounds of 'tradition,' but development nevertheless subsumes these other modes of knowledge under the authority development claims for itself. This authority comes not, as development rhetoric
implies, from the presumably self-evident superiority of the medical solutions
it advocates. Rather, development has authority to the extent that it is able to
make its solutions – whatever they might be – appear self-evident. The language practices of development systematically dismantle a socially animated
local reality, rendering its pattern as a whole inexpressible within development terms. Development appears as a naturally transcendent, necessarily
global institution juxtaposed against limited, fragmented, decontextualised
'local traditions'. It is from this constructed position of transcendence that
development claims the authority and the obligation to provide solutions for
certain societies.

Development discourse presents a certain vision of the way social differ-ence is arranged in the world. In emphasising the difference between 'trad-itional' and 'modern', it removes differences within and between the societies labelled traditional. On this basis development powerfully channels the circu-lation of information. It is through development's mediation that the 'les-sons' from a programme in one country are transported and applied in another. When this happens, it is not a pure 'Western' framework that is being imposed on a given locale in Asia, Africa, or Latin America. Rather, what is transported and put in place, as observed by members of the focus groups and supported by follow-up discussions with, is a model created out of the relationship between the 'modern' and the 'traditional'. (Focus Groups: Ghana, 1991; Malawi, 1991; Malaysia, 1994; Priya, 1997 (telephone inter-view); Ghanaian, Malawian and Malaysian midwives in Oslo, 1996; and Manila, 1999).

For the particular answers development offers to be inevitably the right ones, all local problems must be understood as variations of the same prob-lem. The notion of 'the traditional' is therefore essential to development discourse, as the common denominator of disparate situations that develop-ment can bring under control. Development institutions (and by implication, the interests served through their power) establish their right of entry into local worlds by creating a burgeoning model of modernity.

The authority development (and its experts) has to describe societies, name problems, and propose solutions, comes from the aura of truth that develop-ment agencies present (Escobar, 1988). So, for example, the term 'TBA' appears not only to be efficient but also quite innocent. It is a term that allows varieties of the same kind of practitioner to be conveniently grouped together in development rhetoric. Planners argue that it is necessary to translate from local terms such as those for the many Ghanaian, Malawian and Malaysian forms of 'birth assistance' into more general terms; otherwise, it is said, information about local conditions would be impossible to organise and manage. This, in fact, is exactly my point: without such translations local reality would literally be closed to the power arrangements of development management.

Midwifery knowledge, like other forms of knowledge, is socially con-structed to perpetuate power positions and elite groups. This standpoint advances the belief that there are many 'truths' and that each has equal value to what has been traditionally offered in midwifery education as 'truth'. Dis-ciplines by their very nature profess to represent objective and universal truth and their claim to universalism is only evident because the dominant cultures are, in effect, exporting knowledge-as-truth packaged as a commodity since they have the technical resources to do so. The notion of universalism in this context is not based on shared and agreed perspectives but on an assumption that different groups will either be assimilated into the dominant model or use it as an ideal model for practice. Even if the general aims of the curriculum in economically deprived countries are determined locally, precise curriculum objectives and, moreover, the materials to be used, are on the whole, imported along with specialist consultants to assist in curriculum design and delivery.

The disciplinary context for knowledge production is not 'innocent', objective or value-free. Globally, the disciplines form a power complex mandating particular texts, ways of knowing, and institutional settings as the prime condition for knowledge production. The power of advanced societies such as America and those in Europe over developing worlds has become one based on knowledge production and dissemination.

Making midwives in the modern world: cultural implications for professional programmes

Increasingly midwifery education is moving into higher education institutions and separating itself from the somewhat pejorative image of hospital-based training schools. In all the case study countries midwifery programmes were linked to or embedded in higher education institutions. These programmes are in alignment with the values, beliefs, and status consciousness of mainstream society. They are culturally thought of as the entry criteria for the profession. As a socially valued educational pathway, state and professionally approved programmes carry concomitant benefits, including social recognition and prestige. State-sanctioned midwifery qualifications and awards are the gateway to advanced degrees, which bring prestige, possibly greater remuneration and empower their beneficiaries to practice midwifery, teach new recruits, to effect changes in practice, influence legislation, and to carry out research. In general, it appears that the higher the level of university training of a group of professionals, the higher the social prestige of the entire profession.

While didactic learning is usually primary in universities, midwifery training, like training in other health care professions, always includes some form of preceptorship, in which students are exposed to one-on-one experiential learning with more than one preceptor. Because the clinical parts of university-based midwifery training are mostly carried out in hospitals, students become exposed to and develop expertise in dealing with individuals of diverse sociocultural and economic backgrounds, a wide range of birth complications and unusual health conditions, along with the latest medical technologies. Educators generally work with students to help them develop a critical sense of which technologies have efficacy, under which circumstances, and which ones do not.

A criticism often levelled at university training is that its standardisation stifles individual creativity (Bloom, 1987; Kliewer, 1999). Davis-Floyd (1998) did not find this criticism to apply to the nurse-midwifery students she interviewed in America. In her conversations with them, it was clear that they were accustomed to thinking 'out of the box'. They reported that this kind of unbounded thinking is strongly encouraged by most of their teachers. Nevertheless, a very real problem in university-based nurse-midwifery education is that training offered in large cultural institutions such as universities will inevitably reflect hegemonic philosophies and practices. In the cultural realm of birth, the patriarchal medical model is hegemonic; midwifery training carried out in such institutions will inevitably incorporate many elements of a highly medicalised, patriarchal, and technocratic approach to birth. Thus, midwives will often be required to intervene in birth in ways contrary to the midwifery model in order to successfully graduate and practice.

Concluding discussion: in place of development: dialogue not training

I do not believe that it is a mistake to try to work with women and midwives in other countries. My research has led me to some ideas about what working with midwives could be like. Most importantly, I am convinced that paying lip service to cultural appropriateness is insufficient. I agree with anthropologists that attention needs to be paid to 'local culture' but we need to think carefully about how we pay attention and how we translate cultural understandings of birth. It is important not to generalise about 'tradition' but to talk instead about particular values, situations, and practices as they appear in specific contexts. This requires much more work and knowledge on the part of anyone who would attempt to be a professional expert on midwives and childbirth in many countries. It also requires a different, more holistic kind of research on childbirth.

Generic plans are of limited use, and they can never be a substitute for place and context-specific birth activism. What would a 'training' organised around the understandings of birth in a Ghanaian, Malawian or Malaysian community look like? Moreover, and perhaps more importantly, in multi-ethnic communities what would childbirth look like in perhaps communities of Native American Indian, Afro-American, Asian, Afro-Caribbean, and so on? It would have to be a dialogue, a discussion rather than 'training'. It would not begin with a biomedical model of managed obstetrical care that is then adapted to certain local idiosyncrasies. It would have to begin with the knowledge, values, and concerns of the women involved instead of with the assumptions that their understandings are inadequate and deficient. It would have to take into account the politics of gender and generation in families and the politics of class, caste and ethnic relations in specific communities. It would not necessarily begin by targeting birth attendants in developing countries, but educationalists, academics, researchers and midwives in more advanced societies that peddle their wares abroad.

Biomedicine may have some answers that are good for everyone in the world, but it does not have all the answers. We have to be more humble about biomedical certainties, just as we have to avoid romanticising 'indigenous knowledge' as unequivocally good. Biomedical standards change but the recognition that they do change is often missing when health development efforts take on an evangelical certainty vis-a-vis the practices in non-Western societies. How certain are we about what is 'best'? If developing countries were in a position to rectify North American or European childbirth practices, which of our customs would they most want to alter? A one-way flow of information in development may be harmful to us all.

Chapter 10

The midwifery curriculum

A selection from culture?

In the previous chapter, we considered the cultural implications for midwifery education and practice, which highlighted some of the emerging curriculum issues against the backcloth of a new world order that proclaimed a determination to work for, among other things, common interests, inter-dependence, and cooperation between nations to eliminate gaps between 'developed and developing' countries. The United Nations (1974) stated it would work to ensure accelerated economic and social development to correct inequalities and redress existing injustices, and to ensure peace and justice for present and future generations. These far-reaching objectives set in train a development agenda which, for example, saw the rise of education consultants working with different developing countries to create 'modern' curricula to meet the targets established by the various donor agencies, such as the United Nations, the World Health Organization (see for example, WHO, 1975, 1978, 1986) and the World Bank.

In this chapter I build on the themes raised in the previous chapter and begin to examine the nature of the curriculum as seen in the countries explored. Threaded through the chapter is the continuing theme of cultural types which has been developed further to consider education and curriculum planning from the perspectives of hierarchists, entrepreneurs, isolationists and egalitarians.

Curriculum as a selection from culture: from content and hierarchist perspectives

When asking the question to what extent midwifery knowledge is universal, one has to identify what is common to childbirth in all cultures. In my own illustrations from Africa, Malaysia, America and England, I would argue that not even the birth processes themselves are common and that birth is ultimately a culturally defined activity dependent on the socio-economic and political environment in which it takes place.

Kelly argues that a difficulty arises for those who wish to base decisions about content of the curriculum on considerations of the culture of the society when we attempt to state specifically what that culture is (Kelly, 1989: 36). In modern advanced industrial countries no one pattern of life can be identified as being the culture of that society. Most modern societies are pluralist in nature since it is possible to discern in them a number of different and sometimes conflicting cultures or sub-cultures. Moreover, it is important to recognise that quite apart from sub-cultures being different to each other, most individual members of society will participate in more than one of these sub-cultures at different times or in different aspects of their lives. Thus, not only do most modern societies contain different ethnic groups, each with their own traditions, beliefs, customs and so on, they also contain different religious and social groups, and groups that come together for many different purposes with shared or professional interests, which will have their own norms and cultures.

In developing countries such as Ghana and Malawi, urban centres are becoming increasingly pluralistic. So there is not only the situation for example, in Ghana, where there are more than ninety different tribal groups, all with their own cultural norms, customs and language, but settlers from other countries have moved into the cities to work bringing their own cultures. So we see Asians, Europeans, South Africans, Americans and so on, creating a cultural chop suey. What is of concern is the implication that even if it is believed that the content of the curriculum should be based on culture, it would be impossible to assert with any real expectation of acceptance what that culture is and therefore what the content should be. All that this line of argument achieves is to demonstrate that the curriculum is a battleground of competing ideologies.

The problem is exacerbated by the fact that societies are far from static and this implies that culture is forever in a state of flux. Furthermore, Western cultures are characterised not only by rapid change but also by deliberate change (Taba, 1962: 54). A number of different implications for the development of a midwifery curriculum arise from this.

The first emphasises the impossibility of the task of deciding into which aspects of culture the midwives should be initiated. The second concerns the question about what the relationship of the university, and specifically, the midwifery curriculum, to the greater society should be. Is it the university's role to transmit culture or to transform it? Third, it raises questions about what universities should be attempting to do for their students in a society that is subject to rapid change. Should the university be engaged in skills training or education for lifelong learning? Clearly, in the current phase of rapidly changing social and professional contexts, practitioners need to be equipped to cope with it and even exercise some degree of control. This would suggest that universities should go beyond the notion of initiation of midwives into the culture of the community. To go beyond socialisation and acculturation, to the idea of preparing practitioners for the fact of social change itself, and to adapt to and initiate changes in the norms and values of the community. This requires that practitioners be offered much more than a selection from the culture, even if this could be identified and sufficiently well defined for adequate educational practice. It also suggests that instead of endeavouring to promote in the midwives a body of knowledge, we should be concerned to plan the curriculum to address the capacities we are seeking to develop in them.

If this is the only viable role universities can take in a rapidly changing universe, if we can equip midwives to take their place in society and their chosen profession only by developing in them the ability to think for themselves and make their own decisions, then the question of whether the university is there to transmit or to transform the culture of society has been answered in part. The adoption of such an approach takes the university well beyond the mere transmission of information – a role in a rapidly changing society that would seem untenable. If the university is not itself to transform the culture, it is certainly there to produce people who can and will transform it.

There is another problem that arises if we attempt to establish as part of the content of the midwifery curriculum those things that are regarded as being essentially valuable elements of the dominant culture. This can lead to alienation of some of the students whose experience outside the university may be very different, resulting in a rejection of the education they are offered. This is probably a root cause of the problems of retention in university courses.

This point highlights the weakness of this line of argument since it will be apparent that even if we see it as the task of educators to initiate midwifery students into the culture of society, it would not be possible to offer them the whole of the culture, however defined. A selection would have to be made and, as this is so, any notion of the culture of the society, no matter how acceptable in definition or content, will in itself not provide appropriate criteria for selection. Justification for selection would need to be sought elsewhere. This brings us to the realisation that attempts to base decisions about the content of the curriculum on a consideration of the nature of society are essentially utilitarian arguments that seek a social or sociological justification for curriculum content. This charge can only be avoided if there is an argument put forward that what is valuable in the culture is of universal value, because it has some intrinsic merit that justifies not only its place in the curriculum but also in society itself. Some would argue that there are values that are timeless and transcendental. It is on these grounds that educators argue for inclusion of art, music, literature, values and ideas in the midwifery curriculum. These form a cultural heritage, a human heritage that is universal rather than from any particular nation.

To take this view is, of course, as Kelly (1989: 40) stated, to propound a very different argument from that which seeks justification in the culture itself. It brings us back to the wider question about the nature of knowledge and whether any body of knowledge has or can have intrinsic, objective, absolute value or status. The focus of curriculum content, then, continues to be the nature of knowledge and any curriculum that seeks justification for content in terms that are not utilitarian or instrumental must commence with an examination of the nature of knowledge, which is not unproblematic.

The issues are, therefore, if the curriculum is a selection from culture, then who has the power to make such a selection and from whose culture? As discussed in the previous chapter, in Africa and Malaysia, donor agencies such as the World Health Organization and the World Bank, in giving financial support to developing countries can and do influence internal social, political and health policies. Like ripples on a pond, the Western ideals are impacting on the ways of doing birth in different countries by creating imperatives for measurement, and by imposing modern ideas of time and place of birth. By training practitioners in the mode of Western birth practices, local cultures are conducting birth as perceived to be 'right' way of birth in the Western world.

For a considerable period of time the dominant culture of modernity has been destroying other cultures. In late modernity, however, we are beginning to question some of the values of the earlier era where universalism almost pre-supposed that we could write a curriculum selected from culture because culture was seen as static and science was viewed as 'truth'. But in late modernity, culture is seen to be highly diverse and changing, becoming increasingly 'creole' on the one hand and fundamentalist on the other, with science operating without conclusive 'truth'. What we are seeing is many different cultures operating in different contexts and none can claim to be the conclusive 'reality'. Thus any curriculum based on a selection from culture is one that is based on an idealised version of culture. In curricula concerned with childbirth and midwifery, once we have moved beyond physiology, and that can be disputed as being from a single medico-scientific perspective, arguably little else is universal. We may be able to perhaps distil out a core curriculum but all else is cultural and relating to the ideologies, policies, and discourses of the society.

Have we taken those cultures seriously enough? Let us reflect back to the glimpses of childbirth and midwifery in the country studies. In Africa (chapter 4), Mama Yawa's story and the spirit mediums in Aowin society illustrated the commitment to community, the long-standing relationships with women in the village and the resultant conflict experienced by traditional midwives as they struggled to come to terms with the changing nature of their practice. Flora's story showed how midwifery practice is moving from a community-based activity governed by age-old rituals to modern midwifery practice governed by new rituals. The gown and gloves worn in Flora's story symbolise society's view of childbirth as being dangerous and polluting, as before, but now this was to be contained within the sanitised surroundings of a hospital where women were separated from their communities, family and attendants.

In individualised birth contexts, the midwife is not only isolated from the woman socially, but also emotionally and physically, as midwives increasingly take on roles of control and surveillance, become increasingly specialised in their tasks and align themselves to a production, industrialised model of childbirth. The curriculum is then one that meets the purpose of the role rather than one that meets the needs of women. It is perhaps no longer a selection from culture but a selection from policies established by medical-social and political agendas, influenced by both internal and external forces. In developing countries, those forces may well be represented by agencies such as the World Bank and the World Health Organization.

Of course, for more traditional cultures, creating a curriculum based on a selection from culture may be much easier. The only problem is that the notion of construction of a curriculum is a very Western 'scientific' concept. That is not to say that in traditional cultures, learning is not planned, for in discussion with traditional midwives in Africa, it was clear that they had time-honoured patterns of learning about childbirth. One traditional mid-wife interviewed had been training her niece for more than seven years and she did not consider that she had, as yet, learned enough. The apprenticeship was seamless with working and learning about women, their bodies and how the world around them operated so that birth could happen safely. Moreover, the traditional midwife would only reveal her secrets as and when they were needed, so if the occasion did not demand sharing of information, then it was not shared until the time was right. Thus the initiate learned what was rele-vant to the moment rather than packing a suitcase at the beginning and then being launched off into the world of work on her own.

In this model, which I call the isolationist model of curriculum (figure 10.2, see page 171), the neophyte midwife and the traditional midwife work together as a team, experiencing, sharing and learning as they work with women. For some lay midwives in America this was also the case, particularly among the Amish in Pennsylvania and among the midwives working on the Farm in Tennessee where the experience of childbirth was centred in the community and viewed as a natural part of everyday life, as illustrated by Rachel's story (chapter 7). These communities are separate from mainstream society and thus can develop their knowledge base away from the dominant societal regimes. They work and live as part of the community, and mid-wifery practice becomes a part of everyday life ungoverned by notions of productivity, and demarcation between 'work time' and 'home time'.

The glimpse of Malaysian childbirth and midwifery practice shows the impact of rapidly increasing urbanisation with a concomitant drive for mid-dle-class status in a country where religion continues to dominate cultural forms. Bee's story (in chapter 6) highlighted the move from collective owner-ship of birth at village level to societal ownership of birth at state level. It was the national policies, guided by global imperatives, that were in conflict with the village belief systems that created the problems for Azizah. Malaysia is a country that is striving to be modern and moreover, technologically advanced. A high mortality rate would arguably detract from that image. Consequently, health policies are mainly concerned with reducing mortality and Malaysia has looked to the Western world to provide a model that would assist in this endeavour. The curriculum for midwives is focused on the demarcation between traditional beliefs and modern practices, a move away from birth at home, and away from what might be seen as 'natural' birth to modern birth, hence the comment that 'only peasants squat'.

The model of curriculum adopted clearly lies in the hierarchist arena. The hierarchical model of curriculum (in figure 10.1), leading to state licensing, tends to be dominant in Africa, Malaysia, America and England. In most curricula models the legitimacy of knowledge and practice and the curriculum content, determined by the dominant cultural ideals and policies, were enshrined in hierarchical objectives. The features most commonly seen in state approved midwifery curricula in the case study countries were as follows.

- State regulated curricula were either seen as products and education was instrumental in achieving the required outcome (license to practice,

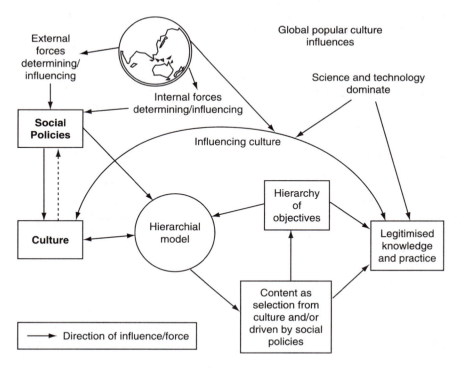

Figure 10.1 Determining forces for curricula design

especially in America), or the curriculum was seen as content and education as the vehicle for the transmission of that content.

- The education and training programmes were time bounded with an emphasis on the quantifiable measurement of achievement of academic and practice outcomes.
- Socialisation into the dominant culture was a prime concern (usually hospital culture with the medical team at the apex of the hierarchy). In Ghana and Malawi, for example, students midwives were required to live in hospital accommodation away from families and friends, thus underlining the liminality of training. They were also expected to wear their white uniforms in the classroom, again emphasising their change in status and separation from their previous lives.
- Emphasis on safety and hospital birth under the control of medical practitioners and an instrumental approach to childbirth were significant features found in all curricula.

The observed outcomes of these common features were:

- a distancing of midwives from women;
- narrowing of women's vision and knowledge about their bodies;
- closing of midwifery mind and narrowing of vision to see only what is legitimised knowledge and practice;
- focus on status creation – fostering opportunities for horizontal violence;
- generation of fear and anxiety among midwives and women;
- change in language (as seen in Africa and Malaysia) which ultimately feeds back into indigenous culture and changes the view of women and their bodies, birth and their children.

In considering the four cultural types, as depicted in figure 10.2, a clear exemplar of the hierarchist approach to curriculum design can be seen in the curriculum as product, education as instrumental model. This is the model most commonly found in America and England and being transmitted to Ghana, Malawi and Malaysia. On investigation in the case study countries, I found that such curricula were generally devised within educational establishments away from the context in which practitioners are required to perform.

A concern with curriculum objectives and, more latterly, learning outcomes has been a striking feature of curriculum planning for many years now. The impetus for this came initially from those who were impressed by the progress of science and technology and believed that the same kind of progress could be made in the field of education if a similar properly scientific approach were to be adopted. As is so often the case, the origins of this movement came from the United States of America. In the United Kingdom

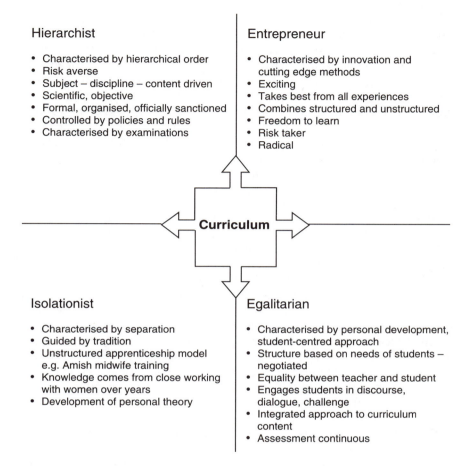

Figure 10.2 Cultural types and the curriculum

and elsewhere, the 'objectives approach' has subsequently been incorporated into midwifery education.

One of the earliest proponents of the objectives movement expressed concern about the rather vague, imprecise nature of the purposes of education and instead claimed that the age of science demanded exactness and certitude (Bobbitt, 1918: chapter 6; Davies, 1976: 47). Bobbitt suggested that teachers should be required to write out their objectives in clear, non-technical language so that students could understand. He also distinguished between what he called 'ultimate' objectives, those for the curriculum as a whole, and 'progress' objectives, those for each class, or in our terms courses, modules, or units, and in addition, for each stage of progress. The cry was taken up by others and in 1924 Charters attempted a 'job analysis' of teaching and offered a method of course construction based on this approach. His suggestion is highly relevant today in that the 'ideals' of education are first identified, then the activities that these involve and finally both are analysed at the level of 'working units of the size of human ability' (Charters, 1924 cited in Kelly, 1989: 51; Davies, 1976: 50). In Charters' view, these small steps need to be mastered one by one and in this way the whole curriculum could be reduced to a series of units and the composite structure could be set out in a chart or graph. This is the model for curriculum modularity today.

This development was accompanied by an interest in testing as a major feature of educational development in the 1930s, and laid the foundations for linking the pre-specifications of objectives and testing of performance. Thus was introduced into educational practice the kind of precise, scientific methods that had begun to yield such dividends in other spheres of human endeavour and especially in industry – so we can see the industrialisation of education, which reflects the current industrialisation of childbirth.

The main characteristic of the 'objectives' approach to curriculum planning was linear and hierarchical sequencing. A classic example of this can be seen in Bloom's taxonomy where the hierarchical nature of the interrelationship of these objectives is fundamental. This is apparent from the graduation of objectives in the cognitive domain away from the acquisition of knowledge of specifics, through such higher-level cognitive abilities as classification, comprehension, application, analysis, and synthesis, to finally acquiring the ability to make evaluative judgements. This was exemplified in the Malaysian curriculum, which demonstrated the division of educational objectives into three domains – the cognitive, the affective and the psychomotor. In the United Kingdom a recent review of the nursing and midwifery curriculum has re-emphasised this approach (United Kingdom Central Council, 2000).

Bloom (1956) in devising his taxonomy also offered another distinction in his division between the head, the heart and the hand – cognitive, affective and psychomotor. I believe that this division between the three domains of knowledge acquisition is perhaps the single causative factor in the so-called theory–practice gap in nursing and midwifery education and practice. The separation of the mind from physical activity in the practice of learning, especially in midwifery, has, I believe, led educators to create separate units of learning. These units comprise either theory or practice, along with separate criteria for assessment of theory and practice, separate evaluative tools and even demarcation in who assesses what. Practitioners more usually assess practice and academics generally assess theory.

More latterly the affective domain in Bloom's taxonomy has generally been ignored since it was and is assumed to be much too difficult to assess. Yet, for midwives, this is a highly significant area for consideration, since childbirth, and consequently an important aspect of the practice of midwifery, is ultimately expressive and concerned with feelings, attitudes and values which science cannot easily have power over. As a result of this dilemma, education and practice have become increasingly instrumental in approach and outcome.

A major contributor to this instrumentation is the fact that the pre-specified objectives are unequivocally behavioural (Kelly, 1989: 57) in nature. Tyler informed us that

> the most useful form for stating objectives is to express them in terms which identify both the kind of behaviour to be developed in the student and the context or area of life in which this behaviour is to operate.
>
> (1949: 46–7)

For Mager (1962: 13) the objectives specify what the learner must be able to do or perform when he or she is demonstrating mastery of the objective. Consequently, the focus of this model of educational planning is on the modification of student behaviour – essentially a reductive process. Success is seen in terms of students being able to demonstrate such modification through assessment of the units of learning. Great store is placed in modular curricula on students demonstrating achievement of the learning outcomes above all else. This has the effect of rendering anything else the student might have learned of lesser importance. There has been increasing evidence in my own experience of the increasingly instrumental view of education in which students will only partake of learning experiences if it leads to a reward for achievement. In modular curricula this relates to the accumulation and transferability of academic credits.

Another feature of the behavioural approach to curriculum design that must be noted here is that, like all scientific approaches to the study and planning of human activity, it endeavours to be value-free. However, childbirth and consequently midwifery practice are steeped in values.

We must consider briefly the main reasons why some people have been and are still concerned to promote this approach. I would concur with Kelly (1989: 60) that there appear to be four reasons for this, which he called the logical, the scientific, the politico-economic and the educational arguments for the use of objectives.

The logical argument claims that part of what it means for an activity to be rational is that it should be directed toward some clear goal or purpose. If education is to be regarded as a rational activity it must state its goals or purposes. The logic of this argument is difficult to deny although it does not necessarily lead to the adoption of a strictly behavioural objectives approach. To state that the curriculum must have purposes is not to say that those must be broken down into the linear hierarchy of behavioural objectives that seems to be essential to this model.

The second main contention that has been offered in support of this model is the scientific argument. This represents an attempt to bring about in education a precision, accuracy and technological efficiency that is admired as the key to advances elsewhere in modern industrialised countries, and thus to render education more respectable in that context. This was clearly the motivation of early exponents of this approach prompted by the application of scientific method to the study of human performance and achievement in industry by men such as Frederick Taylor (Davies, 1976). Promoted by the predominance of behavioural psychology in educational theory in the early years of the twentieth century, this argument increasingly gained a force whose main thrust was to reduce human behaviour to scientific analysis of an essentially means-end ethos and to advocate this methodology to educational planning.

The politico-economic argument is made on a more mundane level but it is one that has become increasingly important through such developments as the national vocational qualification and the competency-based education movement in the UK, so that both its existence and its effects must be clearly recognised. This has extended to higher education with the argument that most educational provision is made at the taxpayers' or employers' expense and they are entitled to a clear statement of what their money is being spent on and what the intended achievements and outcomes are. More importantly and significantly, educational institutions are being called to public and political account for student outcomes in all fields from primary school to higher education.

Finally, some reasons that might be described as educational have been advanced in support of the pre-specification of curriculum objectives. Taba (1962) argued that pre-specified objectives were crucial for evaluation, and that evaluation was in turn crucial for effective teaching. She stated (op cit: 199) 'that those things that are most clearly evaluated are most effectively taught . . . it is difficult to defend the "frills" from current attacks because attainments other than those "essentials" are not readily "demonstrable".' This is a powerful argument if one is prepared to accept the underlying assumptions.

The most fundamental criticism of the objectives approach to curriculum planning is that its attempt to reduce education to a scientific activity, analogous to the processes of industry, commits it to a view of human beings and of human nature that many find unacceptable. For to adopt this kind of industrial model for education, as for childbirth, is to assume that it is legitimate to mould human beings, to modify their behaviour, according to certain clear-cut intentions without making any allowance for their own individual wishes, desires or interests.

This view also assumes that human behaviour can be explored, analysed and explained in the same way as the behaviour of inanimate objects. Furthermore, it assumes that people can be studied scientifically by methods similar to those used by physical scientists or biologists, that their behaviour can be explained in terms of causes rather than purposes, by reference to external forces acting on the individual (i.e. teaching) rather than internal drives and choices of a personal kind.

This passive model of humans is rife in the theory and is not acceptable to those who take the view that people should be regarded as free and active agents in the learning process, responsible for their own destiny and who, as a direct consequence of this, believe it to be morally wrong to deny learners that responsibility and freedom to learn. To approach education in a manner that regards it as an instrumental activity is to lose one essential ingredient that makes education what it is, namely a process whose justification must lie within itself (Kelly, 1989: 83). A curriculum-as-product model of education renders it instrumental and, as a corollary of so doing, often adopts a passive model of human beings. The practice leads to teaching that is more aptly described as instruction or training or even indoctrination, than as education. This ultimately places constraints on both learner and educator that inhibit the freedom of interaction some have claimed to be central to the educative process.

The concern here has not been to argue against the use of an objectives model but to point out its limitations and the implications of its use in an attempt to ensure that those who do adopt this model are fully aware of what that means. An important implication is that an instrumental approach to education must lead to the emergence of a society, or more specifically a midwifery culture, which does not learn, except perhaps by accident, to value things for their own sake. Such a society would be one in which utility is the sole concern, a culture in which all are absorbed only by the means of existence and never by a consideration of its ends. This approach to educational planning has wide-sweeping implications not only for education itself, but also for the nature and indeed the future of society, perhaps even global society and for the attitudes to human life and existence.

Having discussed the purposes of the curriculum we now turn to an exploration of the content of the curriculum and attempt to define from where it should be selected.

The hierarchist model of education: curriculum as content: education as transmission

Many people, from a variety of standpoints, continue to see curriculum merely as content and the process of education as no more than the transmission of knowledge-content assuming that no more is required of the curriculum planner than a list of subjects and a timetable for delivery. This was found to be the case in Africa, America, and many institutions in the UK as well as Malaysia. It is an approach that is simple and clear to policy makers, employers and students alike. Even educators, who one would assume do know better, are increasingly providing a shopping list of 'goods' for consumers of education and training. I would argue that those adhering to this approach would issue from the hierarchist platform (see figures 10.1 and 10.2).

The major weakness in this approach is that at no stage does one find any justification for either the subjects or their content, except in vague and unanalysed phrases such as 'which they need to learn', 'relevant to today's market' or in overtly utilitarian considerations such as 'practical applications' and 'the challenge of employment in tomorrow's world'. We hear of 'bench-marking', of competency targets, graduate outcomes and 'standards', all defined in terms of subject-content and offered as though they are non-problematic. We gain the impression that attempts are being made to 'cash-in' on the some kind of philosophical argument about lifelong learning, fitness for purpose, fitness for practice and fitness for academic award and yet these arguments are nowhere adduced nor are the utilitarian arguments made explicit. To all appearances these definitions are 'plucked from the air' by managers and are complied with by educators.

Justification is needed for any curriculum plan and unless that justification is to be offered only in utilitarian terms some kind of education justification must be provided or at least sought. The lack of justification is the major weakness of the content-transmission model of education. There is little in the model itself that demands of educators a justification for their curricular prescriptions, so that it becomes all too easy to let tradition dictate the curricula for them. Consequently instrumentalism has its own way as the curriculum drifts from one delivery to the next. That is a major problem, as I see it, with a modular curriculum that is fundamentally subject oriented.

The concept of education as transmission or curriculum as content is simplistic and unsophisticated because it leaves out the major dimensions of the curriculum debate and discourages the critical stance that enables the transcendence of the narrower, more specialist perspectives of contributory disciplines. The curriculum should seek to reconcile theory and practice, to look at the actualities of midwifery education from inside, to aspire to praxis so that an attempt can be made to generate a body of theory that has direct relevance for midwifery education and practice. Finally, but most importantly the curriculum must endeavour to seek conceptual coherence and raise questions about the ultimate point and purposes of midwifery practice and not merely those concerning the mechanics of implementation.

Curriculum as content and education as transmission does not raise and cannot raise questions about the purposes of education, unless it sees these merely in utilitarian terms. And this does not encourage midwifery educators to take into account the midwives who are recipients of this content and that process. Their task is to learn what is offered to them as effectively as they can, in the time frame designated. If the effect of the process on them is of any significance this model does not offer any means of evaluating the possible effects beyond assessing the extent of their assimilation of the content. Any other consequences of such learning are beyond the scope of, and relevance to, the model.

It could be argued, however, that it is precisely that effect or these consequences that are at the heart of what might be meant by the term 'education', unless it is to be synonymous with instruction or training. The Malaysian and African curricula make no attempt to disguise their curricula as education since they tend to entitle the course 'midwifery training'. The curricula in both Africa and Malaysia were, at the time of fieldwork, modelled on British curricula of twenty years ago.

Reflecting on distance education

It could be argued that distance education springs from the model of curriculum that is mainly concerned with transmission of content. With regard to the question of how midwifery education designed in the West and transmitted throughout the global village can meet the diverse needs of different countries and localities, I believe the answer lies in the developmental approach to curricula design. In releasing the educational experience from the bonds of a discipline-based orientation, except where it is relevant to the situation under study; in releasing the content of a curriculum from being a selection from the dominant culture and in placing the emphasis on community and individual development, engendering collaboration rather than competition in learning; in being open about the purposes and principles upon which the curriculum is built, I believe that a curriculum designed anywhere in the world could be transportable. The problem with curricula currently designed in the West is the assumption that that is the only way of seeing the world.

Most distance learning materials are designed along the same lines as a traditional curriculum using objectives and standardised content for transmission. As already argued, these approaches fail to address what is important in midwifery education and furthermore may lead to cultural imperialism if transmitted overseas. If a midwifery curriculum is to be transmitted over the Internet, then curriculum planners need to engage in a careful balancing act to avoid overtly or covertly transmitting ideologies whilst being open and sharing information and experiences. The nature of student interaction with the virtual programme is crucial in determining the level of sharing those ideals. Care must be taken to ensure that the sharing is not uni-directional and that the 'exotic' is not romanticised unduly nor the scientific overly valorised.

From personal experience of delivering such programmes over the network, it is clear that the skill of the teacher in avoiding cultural imperialism is as necessary to students at a distance as it is in face-to-face situations in the classroom. The teacher must be able to hold multiple 'truths' to be able to be responsive and challenging to students at a distance. If we are to avoid cultural imperialism, then the teacher cannot be absent, whether in the classroom or over the Internet. But it does beg a question about the teacher's own motives and values in the educational process and the cultural type to which she or he aligns themself.

National policies, influenced by external agencies, are by and large determining curriculum content, what is left out, whose knowledge is legitimate and valid, and what outcomes should be expected from the midwifery course. The result, however, appears not to address issues of equality, such as the sharing of knowledge among the peoples of the world to reduce the gap between developing and developed countries. There seems to be a widening gap between rich and poor, traditional and urban in each country as Bee's story in chapter 5 highlights. The case for broadening the curriculum needs to be made, starting perhaps with an exploration of indigenous knowledge.

The case for indigenous knowledge

A case for situated knowledge that focuses upon the key concerns of women at a local level can be found among the literature concerning indigenous knowledge. It could be argued that the vision of a truly global knowledge partnership might be realised only when the people of the developing countries participate as both contributors and users of knowledge. There is, therefore, a need not only to help bring global knowledge to the developing countries, but also to learn about indigenous knowledge from these countries, paying particular attention to the knowledge base of the rural and impoverished communities. The literature on indigenous knowledge does not provide a single definition of the concept. Nevertheless, several traits broadly distinguish indigenous knowledge from other knowledge.

Indigenous knowledge is unique to a particular culture and society. It is the basis for local decision-making in agriculture, health, natural resource management and other activities. Indigenous knowledge is embedded in community practices, institutions, relationships and rituals. It is essentially tacit knowledge (Polanyi, 1967) that is not easily codifiable but provides the basis for problem-solving strategies for local communities, especially the poor.

Indigenous knowledge perhaps represents an important component of global knowledge on development issues but is so far an under-utilised resource in the development process. Learning from indigenous knowledge, by investigating first what local communities know and have, can improve understanding of local conditions. Moreover, such learning can provide a productive context for activities designed to help communities. Understanding indigenous knowledge may increase responsiveness to clients enabling adaptation of international policies and practices to the local setting that may help improve the impact and sustainability of development assistance. Sharing indigenous knowledge within and across communities may help enhance cross-cultural understanding and promote the cultural dimension of development. Most importantly, investing in the exchange of indigenous knowledge and its integration into the assistance programmes of the World Bank and its development partners may help to reduce poverty.

The integration of indigenous knowledge into the development process, and subsequently the curriculum, is essentially a process of exchange of information from one community to another. Exchange of indigenous knowledge is held as the ideal outcome of a successful transfer and dissemination (World Bank, 1998). This may be seen as essentially a learning process whereby a community from which indigenous knowledge practice originates, the agent who transmits the practice, and the community that adopts and adapts the practice may all learn during the process. It could be argued that indigenous knowledge should play a greater role in the development activities of the World Bank and its development partners. It may, however, lead to the destruction of the very nature of indigenous knowledge itself once it is recorded and catalogued in the way of the Western world.

Curriculum as process and education as development: education through social action and interaction

The development of team midwifery in the United Kingdom has sparked innovative approaches to curriculum design that facilitate the promotion of self-empowerment of midwives, personal efficacy and fosters development of midwives as agents of sustained and effective change. This model would be classified as an egalitarian model of curriculum (figure 10.2). The curriculum in this context aims to be dynamic and interactive drawing on participants' personal theories and experiences in the field, sharing them with their peer group, and fostering an appreciation that all practitioners are expert systems. The academic and practitioners are viewed as equal partners in the venture but recognising that the lecturer has a particular role in spurring them to inquire further, deeper and wider into their knowledge base and experiences. The curriculum follows a philosophically defined structure agreed in partnership with students and other stakeholders.

For Lave and Wenger (1991) participatory education was a way of teaching and learning that enabled practitioners to engage in absorbing and being absorbed in the 'culture of practice'. For them, being absorbed in the culture of practice means both learning and socialisation are part of the process of developing competence in the chosen field of study. As in the examples from both TBAs and the Amish midwives, there is little observable teaching but there is significant learning taking place. For Lave and Wenger, then, a learning curriculum is essentially situated in the context of practice.

Initiate midwives bring with them their own life stories that add to the sum of the practice experience and become a part of the process of situated learning, creating an interaction between the midwife and the social environment of practice. As Kirkham stated:

There is a real sense in which situated knowledge is more complex and more relevant to the care of individuals than conceptual teaching.

(Kirkham, 1997: 191)

As Nelson and Wright (1995) point out, women have multiple dimensions of difference. The complex nature of childbirth ecology, which women and midwives have to negotiate a way through in order to achieve successful and satisfying birth, is underpinned by the interactions between social, emotional, gendered experiences of the life course. The impact of political, economic and legal imperatives, quite apart from the power relations in medically oriented childbirth systems, creates a rich and diverse environment for learning, not only by the initiates but also the women themselves.

One of the main criticisms for the objectives model of curriculum planning was that it assumed a passive model of the individual and considered it appropriate to regard education as concerned with moulding human behaviour according to certain pre-determined goals and blueprints. This must be the case with any curriculum whose prime concern is with extrinsic goals, unless, as Kelly (1989: 93) stated, the person being educated sets those goals.

The starting point in a developmental model of education takes the opposite view of human nature and human potential. It sees the midwife as an active being, who is entitled to control over her or his learning and practice, and consequently sees education as a process by which the degree of such control available to each practitioner can be maximised. All the fundamental underlying principles of the curriculum flow from this standpoint, which is offered not as a scientifically demonstrable theory, but rather as the value position that its advocates adopt and which they recognise as the right of others to reject.

In the developmental model of curriculum, as midwife learners begin to delve deeper into practice and engage in learning conversations with their peers and women in childbirth, they become aware of the need for in-depth understanding of their own and others' worlds. Through this experience they come to recognise the changing nature of practice and appreciate the implications of the compression of time and space that results in the obsolescence of knowledge, leading them to understand the need for continuing learning. They will come to value the opportunities for developing contextually derived meaning in and from practice.

The role of the midwifery lecturer is crucial in the stimulation of critical thought, so it is essential that they become actively involved in the exploration of practice and participate in the research process, becoming both co-researcher and co-subject. The purpose of this approach is to avoid the danger of adopting methods disguised as facilitation and experiential learning that may disguise instrumentalism with a 'human face'. The emphasis on methods and techniques reinforces the notion of theoretical supremacy because of the de-contextualised nature of such approaches. Usher (1992: 12) maintains that we need a critical scepticism and a suitable degree of uncertainty whilst paying attention to the need for a careful deconstruction of theory that arises through practice, theory that arises about practice and the discourses that surround practice, recognising that nothing should be taken for granted.

Jarvis (1992: 246) pointed out that practitioners as learners may encounter a disabling dissonance on return to a structured practice environment governed by the dominant hierarchist culture in which inertia reigns supreme and practitioners and managers may engage in horizontal violence to maintain the status quo (Clements, 1997: 9–14; Leap, 1997: 689) (for literature on horizontal violence, see McCall, 1996 and Skillings, 1992). In these situations the learning and teaching transaction may produce little change as learners are often rewarded for ritualistic and repetitive behaviour whilst experimentation and creativity may be actively discouraged.

> It is really difficult returning to the workplace after attending a course. You get all fired up, find it really stimulating and you go back saying you are going to do something – then nothing happens. Colleagues are not interested in what you have learned – they dismiss your ideas and eventually you give up. There is not a culture of supporting midwives returning from courses – I wonder why we bother sometimes since all most people are interested in is getting through the day.
>
> (Jackie, 1998)

The development of excellence involves a need for generating new cognitive approaches, which will help to effect a perspective transformation, by encouraging the exploration of individual values, beliefs and philosophies. Central to the programme philosophy is acknowledgement that midwives bring their own personal experiences to the learning experience. It is recognised that acceptance of diametrically opposed values of personal versus professional often leads to dissonance within the practitioner. However, as identified by Mezirow (1990) dissonance may pre-empt a change in thinking (perspective transformation), which will ultimately enable the student to 'travel with a different view' (Bass et al., 1999).

The notion of the learning organisation is important here, and particularly so in the context of this curriculum innovation. Crucial to change in practice is the necessity for support for individual practitioners while they come to terms with the changes they are personally going through. Both managers and lecturers have a role to play in this, but for real change to take place, it is necessary to achieve a critical mass of people to carry changes through and to avoid potentially damaging situations for both practitioners and women in childbirth.

If practice is to fundamentally, and not cosmetically, change, then the organisation will need to adopt a learning and experimental ethos, with members acting as learning agents for responding to changes to the internal and external environment, resulting in a process of continuing transformation (Pedler *et al.*, 1991). These transformations can only come about if the symbols that represent childbirth change.

Midwives' stories as vehicles for symbolic exchange: learning from situated knowledge

A major feature of the model of curriculum as process and education as development through social action and interaction, is the use of storytelling as a means of generating symbolic exchanges between midwives both in the UK and overseas. A recent trip to the Farm – a community in Tennessee where women give birth naturally without interventions – facilitated just this type of exchange between the Farm midwives and women, and the British midwives. One respondent informed me that what was clearly evident was the seamlessness of the women and midwives. She reported that during times of storytelling, and sharing information about birth, she could not tell who were the midwives and who were the mothers. Moreover it did not seem to matter. This brings us back to the four cultural types since this model would fit more closely to an egalitarian cultural type and yet it survives because the women and midwives operate outside the dominant medical and social construct of childbirth and midwifery education (figure 10.2).

Perhaps, in order to engage in this form of education for childbirth and midwifery practice, a sanctuary of normal birth has to be created – isolated from the rest, an area where women and midwives can work and learn together. In this model there is no separation between educators and practitioners, they are one and the same. Neither is there a separation between practitioner-teachers and researchers since all three roles are combined in a context of continuous inquiry. The creation of a sanctuary is perhaps to create a liminal space to allow the transition between one form and the next. But unlike liminality as described by Turner (1969), this model represents a transition from one stage of development into the next, like the caterpillar and the butterfly. During this period of change – the liminal phase, there is a need for isolation and distancing from the world.

For real change to occur in childbirth and, as a consequence, midwifery education and practice, there may well be a need to remove midwives and women from the dominant model and the institutions that perpetuate them. There is a need to develop a social model of curriculum that is inclusive rather than exclusive, that addresses the complexity of women's lives within the context of their environment and fosters dialogue and interaction between women, midwives and the various players in the social world.

In summary

In this chapter I have addressed the questions:

- What is the nature of the curriculum and how should it be designed for the future?
- How can midwifery education designed in the West and transmitted over the global network or in educational programmes delivered in the rest of the world meet the diverse needs of different countries and localities?

To answer the question I have explored the differing models of curriculum planning and in so doing have attempted to show the inadequacies identified in the approaches most commonly in use. Criticism of curriculum design from the perspective of its content and the approach through the pre-specification of objectives has led to the emergence of a third curriculum model that requires that we start with an analysis of processes and a statement about procedural principles that are to inform educational practice. This approach, like all others, is not value-neutral but reveals a positive ideological stance and offers a clear basis from which subsequent procedural principles are derived. Of course, the normative and value-laden characteristic of the developmental approach to curriculum design is much criticised, but advocates claim these as major strengths and that in essence all education planning by definition is value-laden and normative and that it is ideological. That being so, the only satisfactory starting point for such planning is in a clear and honest statement about norms, the values, and the ideology from which it is being taken. As Kelly stated:

> Education itself is not a value-neutral process, so that curriculum models based on the idea that is it, or can be, as well as those based on some spurious notion of the objectivity of educational values are at best unsatisfactory because they do not grasp the ideological nettle, or at worst dishonest because they pretend it is not there to be grasped.
>
> (Kelly, 1989: 113)

The egalitarian model reflects more appropriately the role of the teacher in relation to the education of midwives because it fosters an interactive relationship between women, midwives and teachers not least by providing the teacher and student with principles upon which to base professional judgements rather than offering rigid hierarchical frameworks.

Chapter 11

There and back again

The ripples on the pond

I have attempted to illustrate and develop my argument through examples from different times and places. Globalisation, like the ripples on a pond, will naturally have differential effects as it traverses the different parts of the world. But what did globalisation mean to the lives of women in childbirth and the midwives who attend them? Globalisation in the context of this book has been defined as the symbolic exchanges that occur as a result of contemporary engagement with other people in the world through a variety of means that result in exchanges of ideas, beliefs and practices. This led to an exploration of one of the key ideological exchanges – modernity. In the context of childbirth, the globalisation of modernity that includes industrialisation, consumerism, developing markets, and technological advances, has the effect of re-colonising the developing world. These are illustrated through the case studies which attempted to track the symbolic exchanges experienced by women and midwives.

I started with Africa, which, in my view, is the outermost ring of the ripple. Whichever pebble the first world drops in the pond, it always ripples outwards and has an effect, even if it is only a counter ripple in response. In this chapter I explored with women and midwives how globalisation, modernisation and development strategies were changing their daily lives. What I was seeing was not only the physical movement of people towards urban centres but also a movement in thinking and practices among those people who still reside in villages even in the remotest areas of Ghana and Malawi. There appears to be a shift from a traditional, community-oriented worldview to a modern world-view. This appears to be a more profound shift for those people living in urban centres, who have easy access to, or can be easily accessed by, the modern world. So what does that mean for the experience of childbirth? Evidence flowed from women and midwives about how the changes were impacting on them, as I journeyed around Ghana and Malawi gathering stories. I was told about the lives and experiences of traditional midwives, whose stories revealed the increasing symbolic exchange of Western medical ideology that began to overlay and be assimilated into traditional concepts. Traditional midwives were being trained, for example, to observe Western rites of sterility that they found impossible to carry out in their own contexts.

Another story from Africa illustrated the juxtaposition between the herbalist and spirit mediums in one township in Ghana. Here the symbolic movement is away from a community orientation in which the spirit mediums have responsibility within the village to ensure that the whole community is kept healthy, under the guidance of the paramount chief. This means that the mediums, who also act as traditional midwives, not only deal with physical concerns and physical boundaries but also with the spiritual boundaries as well. For spirit mediums, the community is a living organism that is made up of parts, but like a conductor of an orchestra her concerns are with the total 'symphony' not individual instruments. Herbalists, on the other hand, only deal with individuals and do not concern themselves with the community as a whole. Their only concern is looking at the body and the metaphor they used was 'body-as-car' – cars have an engine and if it goes wrong, then the mechanic – the herbalist (or doctor in Western societies) will fix it. The body-as-machine metaphor has reached the very heart of communities in Africa proclaiming the extent of the symbolic exchanges on that continent. Moreover, there is a gender issue since spirit mediums are now mostly women who moved into positions vacated by men who were becoming more exposed to Western ideals through educational opportunities denied to women, and engaged in increased travel and exchange with other herbalists around the country.

Midwifery practice in hospitals was found to have the sediments of modern obstetric rituals in practice during childbirth. One story illustrated the experience of a midwife delivering a woman in an open ward with people walking backwards and forward. There was little attempt to provide privacy, which is a luxury they cannot afford. The midwife wore sterile gloves, she was masked and wearing a green gown and boots but everyone else was walking about without any of those things. Moreover, the midwife went from one woman to the next without changing her 'sterile' garb so one must question whom it was there to protect. The imperative to practise in the style of Western hospitals was strong and yet all the African practitioners had was the knowledge of the scientific ideal, the realisation of what may be required, and that is questionable even within advanced, wealthy societies. But the reality of the situation failed to match this ideal. Consequently, pollution rituals that are being transported from the West are seriously problematic because they define actions that are difficult to achieve in the context of insufficient resources.

Malaysia has experienced a greater degree of the impact of modernisation and indeed, is rapidly modernising and urbanising. Malaysians aspire to achieve the same level of technological revolution as seen in other Far Eastern countries. Once again, similar symbolic exchanges amongst the women and midwives were observed. The Malaysians however, claimed to have achieved more than 90 per cent of births conducted mainly by physicians in hospitals unlike childbirth in Africa where the majority of births occur in rural villages with traditional midwives. The experience of poor women in Malaysia was less than satisfactory in their terms, but they found ways to compensate by engaging a traditional midwife to conduct the various rituals the women still consider important, thus, once again, overlaying the traditional with the modern and vice versa.

In America a considerable number of women experience highly technical childbirth in hospital in spite of attempts to humanise the birth process. From another perspective, an Amish midwife provided a diametrically different concept and approach to childbirth to that of the nurse-midwives. The nurse-midwives interviewed were very committed to normal birth but their definition of what was normal was very different to that seen among the Amish, in that they considered electronic monitoring, intravenous infusion, amniotomy and episiotomy to be normal. The four nurse-midwives in group practice within a small, very wealthy private hospital had been given sanction to deliver women, but realised that they were there on sufferance and so could not 'rock the boat'. Consequently, they had to adhere to hospital protocols to maintain their privileged position. In order to make sense of their practice they were forced to redefine what they did as normal, separating normal from natural birth. Ideologically they did not support natural childbirth. For them, women and childbirth need structure and control.

Obstetric services in Britain succumb to American technological ideology just as other countries and because we are sufficiently wealthy we are better placed to adopt that ideology. Moreover, obstetrics and increasingly midwifery, is enveloped in the all encompassing ideology of childbirth risk. The concept of risk is dominant and powerful and has determined institutional protocols, and the practice and education of both obstetricians and midwives.

What do the stories tell us?

The narratives inform us about the decline of community and the secularisation and institutionalisation of childbirth ritual that is increasingly bound up with technologicalisation and medicalisation. The evidence from the narratives, interviews, observations and content analysis of documentation and curricula reveal the symbolic exchanges of Western approaches to childbirth among women, medical practitioners, health organizations and midwives. This has resulted from a number of key factors that appeared to be influential in these exchanges. These included:

1 Time compression The globalisation of modernity is causing a rupture between internal and external time with external time being compressed and moving further away from internal physiological time frames. The consequence of this is that external time frames are imposed and so induction and acceleration of labour, the ending of a pregnancy that is deemed to have lasted too long and the speeding up of labour to fit some notion of how long labour should last is endemic. Standardisation of labour is now global. The measurement of labour by assessing the dilatation of the cervix and the imposition of the stages of labour to which the woman's body must conform is now almost universal. There is the conviction the cervix only dilates progressively – consequently, there is no recognition that perhaps other factors may impinge and cause a retraction of the cervix. The separation of body, mind and spirit creates disjuncture for women, dislocates them from their body's processes and allows others to dictate what happens in their own bodies, thus disempowering them and creating a loss of control with the consequences of stress, loss of identity and isolation from community and their traditions.

2 Individualism   Moving away from the notion of communal health and increasing individuation.

3 High status   This becomes the goal of urban people (that is, being heard, achieving recognition as a significant part of society, ability to exercise some degree of authority and power over their own, and perhaps others', lives) and is reflected in birthing practices (e.g. will not squat in labour because that is what the peasants do) and breastfeeding practices (bottles are considered more sophisticated and allow more freedom for the woman).

4 Loss of respect for rural people   Rural people, according to one respondent, are considered stupid because they do not have the education of urbanites. Moreover, the urban mind is considered to be harder and less tolerant, tending to ridicule traditions, which is all part of the process of breaking down the fabric of the old world. This is the rhetoric of government that wants to maintain traditional culture and values and yet introduce factors such as finance that increase urbanisation.

5 Language   Changes in language from situated to professional fosters distancing from past, self and community.

6 The inevitability of modernity   Creeps in regardless of attempts to keep it out. Society is changed by mass media, by the influx of people from other cultures for whom various changes have to be made – hotels, shops and their goods, and so on. Local people are required to provide the expected consumer goods and services deemed as necessary. Moreover, researchers, teachers and their ideas, books, journals and other literature, create ripples in the pond also. People travel to other countries, for example, students undertaking education in America or England, are not only changed in themselves, they then carry back ideas and begin to influence changes, however subtly, in their own communities. Even urbanites going into rural areas cause a ripple effect that brings about change. Gareth Morgan (1997) stated that it is the small somewhat inconsequential changes that individuals might bring about that can ultimately result in major change overall (80/20 rule). There is now a critical mass of people who have been exposed to modernity and so it is 'past the point of no return'.

7 Ritualisation of modern technical processes   Antenatal examination; antenatal screening; measurements in labour, etc. If these are done, the baby will be all right. Training in Malawi, Malaysia and Ghana results in the replacement of old rituals with new, which could engender a false sense of security.

8 Disorientating dilemmas for traditional midwives   TBA training may well begin a de-skilling process as traditional midwives are exposed to Western methods and practices. Over time traditional knowledge and skills will be lost and they will not be able to pass them on to their apprentices, thereby eliminating a whole knowledge base – again distancing women from their history. Moreover, forceful dictates from the West that conflict with traditional beliefs and values often lead to disorientation, confusion and perhaps resistance.

9 Technologicalisation becomes an important tool in the process of star-making   Adds to the drama of the situation, adds to the complexity ratio. Midwives chase this dream too – the more complex, the better and more proficient they seem, the bigger stars they are.

10 Medicalisation and medical oppression   The medicalisation of childbirth.

11 Doctor as culture hero

> If doctors see themselves as the star and that status, power reinforces their sense of self, personal identity, and value and midwives see themselves as the star for the same reason, how do the women see themselves? It depends on to whom they relate their story – to have a baby in hospital with all the high tech equipment and doctors dancing attendance on one – sounds like stardom in the village – but privately, she may well feel like an appendage – if she is noticed at all and may well see the doctor as the star. There must be a difference in urban and rural areas and this must also depend on their cultural type also. The consumption of stardom.
>
> (Karrie, a midwife, UK, 1997)

Figure 11.1 summarises the trends and counter-trends in global symbolic exchanges associated with advanced societies and the influences and lessons from developing societies.

Dominant trends from advance technological societies	Counter trends from advanced technological societies
• technological scientific medicine • 'death-as-enemy' metaphor is used to drive increased surveillance • stethoscopes and white lab coats, masks, theatre garb as symbols of authority and power • language exclusive; research and measurement as dominant ideologies, mainly conducted by advanced societies • emphasis on time and control through monitoring and measurement • individualistic; blame rests on individual • isolated from community – emphasis on birth in hospital • state takes control away from family through legislation • diagnosis rests with doctor • systems of experts and specialists	• partnership between women and midwives as symbol of shared power • language inclusive; emphasis on communication and shared language • research considers what is important not just what is measurable • emphasis on physiology • community and family oriented; shared decision-making • women take control of childbirth experience • women become expert systems in their own childbirth • midwives as earth mothers?

Influences from East and South

- traditional medicines – indigenous knowledge
- community oriented – holistic but also individual – blame for individual ills rests with cosmos
- community implicated as well as individual in ill health

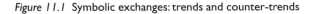

Figure 11.1 Symbolic exchanges: trends and counter-trends

Concerning cultural types and myths of nature

I explored the concept of the medically defined obstetric risks that generate fear in people for many different reasons. When I returned to look at my cultural types model, I saw that the midwives and women I had engaged with fell into all four, or perhaps five cultural types.

As discussed earlier, there are the hierarchists who believe in structure and organisation; the egalitarians (I like to call them 'checo-warriors' (childbirth eco-warriors)), who subscribe to partnership and campaign for better childbirth for women; the isolationists, who separate themselves from the dominant organisational culture and its protocols; the entrepreneurs, who are creative risk takers and who work mostly on their own trying innovative schemes to bring about change; and another type that I define as ritualists. These people may be found both among traditional midwives in rural areas of developing countries and conventional midwives in the most advanced societies – the metaphor that best describes them perhaps is 'just in case'. Perhaps what determines ritualist actions is fear and that fear emerges from a feeling that regardless of whatever information one might have that is contrary to your deep-seated anxieties, you have to engage in the ritual just in case it all goes wrong. In this way it is almost like a belief in some mysterious force that will punish you if you fail to pay the correct tribute. These feelings were exhibited among midwives in every country and among medical practitioners and women also. When asked why particular practices were still conducted despite evidence refuting their validity, the reply was often 'well yes I know all that but I still do it just in case'. This was the answer given by a traditional midwife regarding putting cow dung on the baby's cord. Many would explain that as simple ignorance, but when questioning midwives in a group who were undertaking an advanced degree, the response was the same only in a different context with a different set of practices that had likewise been discredited. Perhaps these rituals work to anchor them to their firm belief systems and to a sense of stability and continuity and this works for both beneficial and detrimental rituals.

Clinging to some rituals may also be part of some notion of expertise, professional or non-professional. Expertness comes from what you know and how you practise and perhaps this clinging is a concern about relinquishing that. The rituals, whether conducted by the traditional midwife in the village or the professional nurse-midwife in the hospital, are perhaps maintained to reinforce power positions. Rituals serve to define the span of control, only the practitioner has the authority and power to conduct the ritual, as in the example from Malaysia, where the traditional midwife is the only person who can conduct all fourteen rituals surrounding childbirth. This is in contrast to the professionally trained midwife who can only conduct four of them. The powerful position is difficult to relinquish since as soon as they are challenged to give up rituals, in effect they are being forced to de-'professionalise' at that level.

> In terms of childbirth this may not be a bad thing because women should be with women on an egalitarian level. We have been questioning ourselves about whether we have the notions of professional right anyway and even with midwife teachers and students, it is not an equal partnership and should we be reinforcing what is professional behaviour rather than talking about what it should be to be a woman with a woman in this time of ecstasy. Those rituals are also bound up with what it is to be a professional with power and control. But some rituals are also good rituals. You tend to think of ritualistic behaviour as being people who don't question what they are doing but we also see good rituals where people come in from a perspective which we saw in Tennessee which was a ritual of non-interference, completely standing back, the birth area is

sacred – that was a ritual. They went for a real dance making this place sacred – that was a good ritual, so it works on both levels.

(Fran, British midwifery lecturer, 2001)

Together, the case study chapters provided a platform from which to explore the social and cultural implications for the education of midwives and further development of the myths of childbirth model in the context of education. The myths of childbirth are concerned with our concepts of where we place the nature of women's bodies in relation to childbirth, on the continuum of being robust to being completely fragile. Such placing determines the way we approach practice, the way we approach education and the way we approach childbirth itself as women. Therefore if a person comes from a hierarchist perspective she believes that birth needs to be structured. It needs to be conducted in a hierarchical power structure with people at the bottom 'doing as they are told'. This is the same in education, where there are exams, tests and assessment and there is a body of knowledge that the teacher transmits to students who are passive. If a person comes from an egalitarian point of view, the structure is negotiated and shared. Knowledge comes from a variety of different sources, it is all examined for its merits, and some knowledge is rejected and other knowledge is accepted. Therefore the myths of childbirth are quite important in terms of where people choose to place themselves in the system.

In America there are different models of learning ranging from apprenticeships, that adhere to a model of learning rather than a model of education and formal curricula that prepare midwives, to masters' degree level. The latter tend to undertake their preparation in a hierarchist institution that conforms to a model of education, which is defined, structured, tested and validated in universities. So where we place ourselves in terms of learning midwifery is interesting. In Britain, of course, there is no choice; the profession of midwifery has placed itself in the hierarchist model. Alternative models of education and curriculum are strongly discouraged, and practice is tightly controlled by institutions. This is ultimately leading to a closing of the mind, a narrowing of the experience.

You also get a closing of the minds because in the end it becomes so scientific and when you are trying to match the scientific body of evidence with something as natural as childbirth you realise they don't match. You actually start to think that you are the one who hasn't got the answers and you try to compete with a scientific body of knowledge. You can't trust your intuition, you can't trust watching, observing, touching – you can't trust those ways of knowing so you start to identify more with the scientific body of knowledge which becomes even bigger and better and more advanced than you could possibly be. The average person couldn't keep up with it so in effect you start to close your mind. You actually start (not deliberately) to identify with the scientific paradigm.

You are persuaded that this is the right way and that what you see, feel and hear from women is the wrong way and you actually then block yourself off to all the other ways of knowing which make sense to you. You then find that it is incredibly difficult to maintain your good intentions to listen to women. But you have to identify with one and because we work in a culture where the emphasis is on the scientific, technical, and rational, these are generally chosen as the right ways of knowing. We work in a culture where the profession and society sets great store by that and our personal knowledge becomes secondary or irrelevant. This causes real tension because I believe that most midwives in their hearts are finding it difficult to marry the two together which is why they are having to reject one or the other and what they reject, unfortunately, is their intuition and women's wisdom.

(Fran, British midwifery lecturer, 2001)

This way of thinking, practising and educating is spreading across the world and is beginning to be dominant even in the smallest communities under the conditions of globalisation. But the interesting thing that is happening under those same conditions is that we now have a spin-off from the fact that women and midwives are using the World Wide Web and Internet to communicate with each other in a way that was denied to them before. The route for accessing authoritative and legitimised knowledge was through hierarchical institutions of education and service. Practitioners and women had to go through that process of education to access information about childbirth generally and the only other information was that of pseudo-scientific, folklore science mediated by the popular press that would fashion the information according to their social and political stance. Nowadays with the technology that is increasingly available women, midwives, lay midwives, and anybody with an interest, can share information, rally support and explore other ways of birth from different cultures. I would argue that through the use of the Internet a community of women and midwives is developing that is global in scale and exists in real time. This community of midwives and a global community of women have and can share knowledge and wisdom that is different to the dominant medical paradigm.

The impact of the global network works in two key ways that are generating global data on childbirth knowledge as midwives and women increasingly share personal theories they had not written about or were not legitimised through publication. These practitioners and women are finding a way of subverting the dominant elite who control the professional publications, who only accept articles that are within the dominant mode. As midwives and women write their stories and share their experiences, there is an emerging form of alternative legitimation. Previously midwives' knowledge was secretly shared in the coffee room over cups of tea or in the corridors. It was rarely wider than that, so there appears to be a significant level of symbolic exchange occurring. Exploring the Internet revealed more than fifty different web pages concerned with childbirth and midwifery that can be accessed by anyone with an interest, which may ultimately bring about a major shift in the ways women and midwives think about childbirth. Women are going to be as informed, if not more so, than the midwives and obstetricians who are supposed to be the 'expert systems'. Women will become their own expert systems to a certain extent and will be well placed to challenge the dominant medical view. Ultimately, the body of knowledge will then become shared and perhaps a common language will be developed.

Despite this potential shift in access to knowledge, the possible contribution to women's knowledge and experience may remain trapped among their group, and still not be considered authoritative or legitimate by the medical fraternity. Childbirth is placed firmly in the medical-curative domain that mobilises potent symbolic capital.

Western doctors as well as traditional healers globally manipulate symbolic media that connects the physical with the social order (Comaroff, 1982: 52). In the face of the fear and anxiety that often accompany infirmity, curative processes powerfully reinforce the logic of inherent meanings and implicit images of self and their context drawn from the wider cultural system. Medicine reaches down to the very heart of the deep-seated paradoxes of the human condition which childbirth lays bare, harnessing the physical symbols through which these are expressed with values reflecting specific concerns. Returning the woman to 'normal' thus reaffirms the integrity of an implicit construction of reality and its enveloping symbolic order. Tangible medical knowledge provides the explicit rationale for this process, presenting as 'natural' what is actually a culturally constituted and socially motivated image of childbirth (after Figlio, 1976: 17–35). Childbirth often heightens awareness of more fundamental dilemmas not adequately addressed in particular healing processes, but fundamental to social relationships. Affliction may thus lead to more comprehensive 'dis-ease' within the social system itself. This is just as it is seen by the Aowin spirit mediums in Ghana who view dis-ease as much of an affliction of the community as the individual.

As a discrete body of knowledge and technique, medicine has become progressively disengaged from the language of cosmology and morality, from a system of knowledge addressing the relationship of between human beings, and from nature and spirit. In the dialectical process of modern history, the fragmentation and the progressive disengagement of spirit and matter have reinforced and been reinforced by the rise of empiricism and industrial technology and have spread symbolically through the processes of globalisation. Consequently we have seen a shift from traditional ideas about childbirth to modern beliefs, ideologies and values represented in a shift in allegiances towards hierarchical values and practices among midwives, and women (see figure 11.2). For the language of childbirth globally has become part of the circumscribed discourse of science, designed to exclude from its frame of

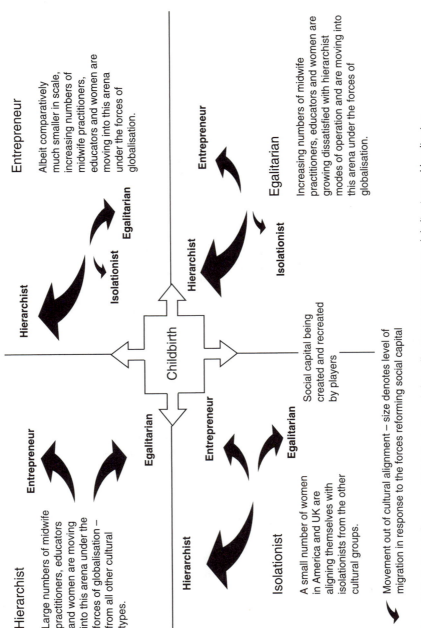

Hierarchist

Large numbers of midwife practitioners, educators and women are moving into this arena under the forces of globalisation – from all other cultural types.

Isolationist

A small number of women in America and UK are aligning themselves with isolationists from the other cultural groups.

Entrepreneur

Albeit comparatively much smaller in scale, increasing numbers of midwife practitioners, educators and women are moving into this arena under the forces of globalisation.

Egalitarian

Increasing numbers of midwife practitioners, educators and women are growing dissatisfied with hierarchist modes of operation and are moving into this arena under the forces of globalisation.

Social capital being created and recreated by players

Movement out of cultural alignment – size denotes level of migration in response to the forces reforming social capital

Figure 11.2 Cultural types and childbirth choices: shifting allegiances in response to globalisation and localisation

reference all unspecific references, and closing off areas of women's lives irrelevant to its particular concerns.

Yet through personal experience, especially in childbirth, women disconcertingly challenge the adequacy of tacitly assumed material individualism and some are shifting allegiances toward more egalitarian modes of operation or, indeed, are isolating themselves to achieve their personal goals (see figure 11.2). At such times they come face to face with universal conundrums of human existence as they are refracted through the lens of their sociocultural system and projected in such contexts as that of childbirth practice (after Comaroff, 1982: 58). Childbirth stresses the ambiguities of physical and social being, and of life and death, as urgently as any other human experience, and women more often than not look for the resolution of dilemmas in medical processes. Americans, in particular, are caught within the contradictions of their own sociocultural order. The ideology of individualism that is a feature of their national identity, rests upon the reinforcement of the symbolic oppositions which in childbirth they sense and try to transcend. Thus, with an alienated image of self, caught in the opposition of mind and body and cut adrift from the wider social and moral context, they attempt to impose 'meaning' upon an estranged world.

There is evidence to suggest that the dependence of the sick upon others, whether with or without special skill, engenders ambivalence in most cultures (Illich, 1976). But the extreme dependence upon specialist knowledge and professional intervention which has developed in modern Western societies has led to considerable popular dis-ease – although it has not really led to such consciousness as would make it possible to confront the contradictions upon which the dissonance is based. Indeed, the conditions for the development of such consciousness within the logic of scientific-technological culture was the subject of considerable debate among students of ideology (see Habermas, 1971: 111; Mandell, 1980: 501; Marcuse, 1972: 138). Moreover, what is deemed scientific by the public and policy makers in government is often folklore science, pseudo-science that has been translated by the popular press for public consumption. In this way the true details of the scientific results are distorted and disseminated to a larger audience who have little or no access to the full research papers. Furthermore, it seems that as each scientific theory is abandoned for the next by scientists, this is not the case with either the popular press or the policy makers who cling to old studies while adding new data creating a mismatch of information on which it is often inappropriate to base decisions about health care, lifestyles or childbirth practice. It is this confused data that is being distributed globally through media networks and the world wide web.

Our inability to come to terms with childbirth systems failure stems from the fact that television reduces political discourse to sound bites and academia and medicine organises scientific and intellectual inquiry into narrowly specialised disciplines. As a result we become accustomed to dealing with complex issues, such as childbirth, in fragmented components. Yet in the complex world in which we live nearly every aspect of our lives is connected in some way with every other aspect. Consequently, if we limit ourselves to fragmented approaches to dealing with universal problems or natural physiological events such as birth, it is not surprising that our solutions prove inadequate. If human beings are to survive the predicaments we have created for ourselves, a capacity for whole-systems thought and action must be developed. Whole-systems thought must include the environment, culture, politics, issues of power and control, institutions and so on.

> Whole-systems thinking calls for a scepticism of simplistic solutions, a willingness to seek out connections between problems and events that conventional discourse ignores, and the courage to delve into subject matter that may lie outside our direct experience and expertise.
>
> (Korten, 1995: 11)

Reflecting on the research

What I learned was that my experiences and that of others do not fit comfortably into suitably defined and labelled boxes marked medicine, body, mind, economics, environment, social, cultural, science, magic and so on. Women and their experiences of childbirth continually evade the boundaries that have been demarcated by obstetricians, policy makers, insurance agencies and midwives who fall into a hierarchist mode.

The broader framework of contextual issues surrounding the multi-dimensional study directed me to an extensive examination of the literature regarding modernisation, globalisation, economic and structural reform, sustainable development, environmental issues, sociocultural factors, economic imperatives and the role of global corporations in determining the lives of women in childbirth. The study has enabled me to look at the impact of symbolic exchanges on women and midwives and challenged me to consider safe motherhood and midwifery education and practice in this context.

I consider that the greatest strength of this study was not only its breadth and depth, but also that it was undertaken in the cultural context. I was privileged to work with women and midwives at every level of those societies under study – from government to village levels.

It is acknowledged that this is a highly complex and ambitious research project. To address issues of childbirth in one country would have been deemed courageous but to consider childbirth in five countries on four continents was perhaps, on reflection, foolhardy. The sheer quantity of data alone was daunting and proved difficult to control at times but the validity of the research, I would argue, did not come from the volume, but from the multi-perspective and multi-dimensional approach adopted in engaging with women, midwives and birth attendants in five countries.

Consequently, the validity comes from veracity rather than numerical calculations.

What could have been perceived as a weakness of the study, that my primary purpose for being in Malaysia and America was to enact another role, became, in the end, a strength. Despite finding myself constrained to specific areas of those countries rather than having the freedom to travel more widely to collect data, my role as an educator teaching research, developing curricula and meeting students and staff also had the effect of opening avenues for study, and access to materials and participants that might have otherwise been denied me. For example, it would not have been a simple matter for me to access the Amish community without the assistance of the nurse-midwives in Pennsylvania.

Another fundamental weakness of the research was my own lack of local languages. The fact that I had to rely on translators in Africa and Malaysia caused its own challenges and difficulties. It was not always possible to check out my interpretations with the women involved at the time or in some cases later since many of the interpretations came after I had left the country. Moreover, lacking sufficient insight into local customs meant that I had to rely heavily upon local midwives for guidance. This was both a weakness and a strength since the approach taken by the local midwives was one of enfolding me into the community. I was 'adopted' in Africa as one of their own – lost to the New World (since I am West Indian) – and they considered that I had to be re-integrated into their community. Consequently I learned a great deal more, perhaps, than I would have otherwise and gained access to ceremonies and births that an outsider would have had to spend much longer with the various groups to achieve. This, in the long run, allowed me to gather ethnographic data in a much shorter time frame than is usual. It is clear, however, that much longer periods of time need to be spent with selected groups of women and midwives in different countries to truly delve deeper beneath the surface of what could be, in effect, only superficial changes. One possible research question would be to what extent resistance to Western ideology exists and how this is manifested globally. I would be interested, for example, to explore to what extent resistance in developing countries, if it exists, mirrors resistance in Western countries.

This book is my story and recording the data and writing the book itself meant that I had to make a selection from field notes for analytical purposes and then a further selection to provide illustrative material to illuminate the thesis. Any research of this complexity will entail a double selection process from data, even if it is not acknowledged, and may in itself present an aspect of subjectivity in the writing.

I found the storytelling approach to be unequivocally valuable. It allowed me to access areas of women's lives as well as my own life, to make sense of the experience. Maintaining a daily diary permitted me to take a heuristic approach to the study since this became for me a personal, as well as a professional journey. Personal bias, of course, played a significant part in the research, yet the breadth of the study and depth of the experience, I believe, compensated for any indulgences that I might have engaged in. The danger was one of not seeing the obvious, both on the part of the participants and the researcher. It would have been all too easy to see the poverty in Africa and Malaysia and been swept away with the deficiencies in childbirth systems and yet maintain a balanced view of the people and their struggles. The Africans I met struggled – but mainly overcame difficulties with ingenious inventions. The American nurse-midwives faced their own challenges and had novel solutions. In attempting to maintain honesty in the research I used a technique of interplay of stories – juxtaposing one set of issues against another to 'see' from different perspectives. This enabled me to avoid falling into the trap of exoticism.

Participants' responses, some may argue, could well have been only what they thought I wanted to hear. This was especially a concern in Malaysia where it is considered impolite to disagree with a 'guest' or teacher, or with someone they considered further up the hierarchical ladder. I found that the telling of stories helped considerably with this aspect. I was not asking direct questions to which respondents were required to 'tell the truth'; I was inquiring about their lives as they chose to explore themselves through stories.

The symbolic exchanges impinging on women's lives and midwives' practices as a result of globalisation, as revealed in their narratives of childbirth, point to a lost world where some of the premodern practices may be considered more valuable than current ones. Perhaps late modernity is allowing us to more clearly identify them. Too often life is dominated by economics, politics and technology, and this book attempts to demonstrate how these dominate childbirth. But more fundamentally it is about the importance of human social needs, and the way childbirth is affected by the growing conflict between the economic systems, technological advances, and medical dominance, and the fulfilment of our social needs. The book's main message is of the primary importance of social relations to women in childbirth, whether rich or poor – the quality of social relations has been a prime determinant of the experience of childbirth and the quality of life.

Bibliography

Abercrombie, N. (1990) *The Dominant Ideology*. London: Heinemann.

Abercrombie, N., Hill, S. and Turner, B.S. (1980) *The Dominant Ideology Thesis*. London: Allen and Unwin.

Abercrombie, N., Warde, A., Sayer, A. and Walby, S. (2000) *Contemporary British Society*. (3rd edn). Bristol: Polity.

Abrahams, R.D. (1973) 'Ritual for fun and profit (or the ends and outs of celebration)'. Paper delivered at the Burg Warnenstein Symposium 59, Ritual: Reconciliation in Change. Cited in R. Davis-Floyd (1992), *Birth as an American Rite of Passage*. Berkeley, Calif.: University of California Press.

Abu-Lughod, L. (1990) 'The Romance of Resistance: Tracing Transformations of Power Through Bedouin Women'. In Peggy Sanday and Ruth Goodenough (eds), *Beyond the Second Sex: New Directions in the Anthropology of Gender*. pp. 313–337. Philadelphia, Pa.: University of Pennsylvania Press.

Adamson, P. (ed.) (1996) Commentary: A Failure of Imagination: The Progress of Nations: Women 1996 Report. UNICEF.

African Indigenous Science and Knowledge Systems (1999) *http://members.aol.com/Afsci/africana.htm*

Aharoni, Y. (ed.) (1993) *Coalitions and Competition: The Globalization of Professional Business Services*. New York: Routledge.

Akinware, M.A. and Ojomo, A.A. (1993) 'Child Rearing Practices and Their Associated Beliefs in Nigeria: A Paper Based on the Baseline Studies Conducted in Five Local Government Areas in Nigeria UNICEF (1987–1990)'. Paper presented at the Workshop on Child-rearing Practices and Beliefs, Windhoek, Namibia, October 26–29, 1993.

Albrow, M. (1996) *The Global Age: State and Society Beyond Modernity*. Cambridge: Polity.

Alexander, J. (1990) 'Mobilizing against the State and International "Aid" Agencies: "Third World" Women Define Reproductive Freedom'. In Marlene Gerber Fried (ed.), *From Abortion to Reproductive Freedom: Transforming a Movement*. Boston, Mass.: South End Press.

Alonso, A.M. (1992) 'Gender, Power, and Historical Memory: Discourses of Serrano Resistance'. In J. Butler and J. Scott (eds), *Feminist Theorize the Political*. Boulder, Colo.: Westview Press, pp. 404–425.

Anderson, L. (1998) Human Capital in the Social Sciences. *Items – Social Science Research Council*, 52(2–3): 31.

Annandale, E. (1987) 'Dimensions of Patient Control in a Free-standing Birth Center'. *Social Science and Medicine*, 25, 1235–48.

Appadurai, A. (1990) 'Disjuncture and Difference in the Global Cultural Economy'. *Public Culture* 2(2): 1–24.

Apps, J. (1988) *Higher Education in a Learning Society*. San Francisco: Jossey-Bass.

Armstrong, D. (1983) *Political Anatomy of the Body*. Cambridge: Cambridge University Press.

Arney, W.R. (1982) *Power and the Profession of Obstetrics*. Chicago: University of Chicago Press.

Arnold, H. (ed.) (1994) *William Corbett: A History of the Protestant Reformation*. (abridged). London: Fisher.

Atkinson, P. and Heath, C. (1985) *Medical Work: Realities and Routines*. Aldershot: Gower.

Audit Commission (1997) *First Class Delivery: Improving Maternity Services in England and Wales*. Oxon: Audit Commission Publications.

Ayres, L. and Poirier, S. (1996) 'Virtual Text and the Growth of Meaning in Qualitative Analysis'. *Research in Nursing and Health*, 19: 163–169.

Bader, M.B. (1979) 'Breast-Feeding: The Role of Multinational Corporations in Latin America'. In V. Navorro (ed.), *Imperialism, Health and Medicine*. New York: Baywood.

Balaskas, J. (1991) *New Active Birth*. London: Thorsons.

Balaskas, J. and Balaskas, A. (1983) *New Life: The Book of Exercises for Childbirth*. London: Sidgwick and Jackson.

Banik, B.J. (1993) 'Applying Triangulation in Nursing Research'. *Applied Nursing Research*, 6(1): 47–52.

Banks, A.C. (1999) *Birth Chairs, Midwives and Medicine*. Jackson, Miss.: University Press of Mississippi.

Barker, C. and Turshen. M. (1986) 'Primary Health Care or Selective Health Strategies'. *Review of African Political Economy*, 36: 78–85.

Barthes, R. (1973) *Mythologies*. (trans. Lavers, A.) Boulder, Colo.: Paladin.

Barrett, J.F.R., Jarvis, G.J. and MacDonald, H.N. *et al.* (1990) 'Inconsistencies in Clinical Decisions in Obstetrics'. Lancet 336: 549–551.

Baudrillard, J. (1994) *Simulacra and Simulation*. (trans. Sheila Faria Glaser). Ann Arbor, Mich.: University of Michigan Press.

Bass, J. *et al.* (1999) BSc(Hons) Midwifery – unpublished curriculum document.

Beattie (1987) 'Making a curriculum work'. Cited in P. Allen and M. Jolley, *The Curriculum in Nursing Education*. London: Croom Helm.

Beauchamp, T.L and Childress, J.F. (1994) *Principles of Biomedical Ethics*. New York: Oxford University Press, 1979 (4th edn).

Beck, U. (1992) *Risk Society: Towards a New Modernity*. London: Sage.

—— (1999) *World Risk Society*. Cambridge: Polity.

—— (2000) *What is Globalization?* Cambridge: Polity.

Bellah, R., Madsen, R., Sullivan W.M., Swidler, A. and Tipton, S.M. (1985) *Habits of the Heart: Individualism and Commitment in American Life*. Berkeley, Calif. University of California Press.

Belmont Report (1979) The National Commission for the Protection of Human Subjects of Biomedical and Behavioral Research, 'The Belmont Report: Ethical

Principles and Guidelines for the Protection of Human Subjects of Research, OPRR Reports', April 18, 1979.

Benoit, C. (1991) *Midwives in Passage: The Modernisation of Maternity Care* (Social and Economic Studies, 44). Canada: Inst. of Social and Economic Research.

Bergstrom, S. (1996) 'On the Sustainability of Maternal Health in the Debt Trap'. Paper presented at the ICM 24th Triennial Congress, Thursday 30th May, Oslo, Norway.

Beynon, C.L. (1988) ' "Striving to better oft we mar what's well" . . . Management of Normal Labour'. *Midwives Chronicle*, Sept 101(1208): 280–289.

Blank, R. (1994) *Voices of Diversity*. New York: Amacom.

—— (1999) *Voices of Diversity: Real People Talk About Problems and Solutions in a Workplace Where Everyone Is Not Alike*. Boulder, Colo.: Netlibrary, Inc. *http://www.netlibrary.com/summary.asp?ID=2455*

—— (2000) *From the Outside In: Seven Strategies for Success When You're Not a Member of the Dominant Group in your Workplace*. New York: Amacom.

Bloom, A. (1987) *The Closing of the American Mind: How Higher Education has Failed Democracy*. New York: Simon and Schuster.

Bloom, B.S. (1956) Taxonomy of Educational Objectives: the Classification of Educational Goals. New York: David McKay.

Bobbitt, F. (1918) *The Curriculum*. Boston: Houghton Mifflin, ch.6.

Bolton, G., Rowland, S. and Winter, R. (1990) 'Writing Fiction as Enquiry into Professional Practice'. *Journal of Curriculum Studies*, 22(3): 291–293.

Bolton, P., Kendall, C., Leontsini, E. and Whitaker C. (1989) 'Health Technologies and Women of the Third World'. *Women and International Development Annual*, 1: 57–100.

Bowles, N. (1995) 'Storytelling: A Search for Meaning within Nursing Practice'. *Nurse Education Today*, 15(5): 365–369.

Boyne, R. (1990) 'Culture and the World System'. In M. Featherstone (ed.), *Global Culture*. London: Sage.

Brackbill, Y., Rice, J. and Young, D. (1984) *The Legal Low-Down on High-Tech Obstetrics*. St Louis: C.V. Mosby.

Brodie, P. (1996) Being with women: the experiences of Australian team midwives. (unpublished thesis). Sydney: University of Technology.

Brown, J., Collins, A. and Duguid, P. (1989) 'Situated Cognition and the Culture of Learning'. *Educational Researcher*, 18(1): 32–42.

Brown, M.M. and Jolly, R. (1999) *Human Development Report 1999. Globalization with a Human Face*. New York: United Nations Development Programme.

Bruner, J. (1991) 'The Narrative Construction of Reality'. *Critical Inquiry*, 18: 1–2.

Brunn, S.D. and Leinback, T.R. (eds) (1991) *Collapsing Time and Space: Geographic Aspects of Communication and Information*. London: Routledge.

Bryman, A. (1992) 'Quantitative and Qualitative Research: Further Reflections on their Integration'. In J. Brannen (ed.), *Mixing Methods: Qualitative and Quantitative Research*. Aldershot: Avebury, pp. 57–78.

Burgess J. (1996) 'Focusing on fear'. *Area*, 28 (2): 130–36.

Bury, M. (1982) 'Chronic illness as biographical disruption'. *Sociology of Health and Illness*, 4: 167–182.

Busia, K.A. (1954) 'The Ashanti of the Gold Coast'. In Daryll Forde (ed.) *African Worlds: Studies in the Cosmological Ideas and Social Values of African People*. London: Oxford University Press.

Butterworth, T. and Bishop, V. (1994) 'Identifying the Characteristics of Optimum Practice: Findings from a Survey of Practice Experts in Nursing, Midwifery and Health Visiting'. *Journal of Advanced Nursing*, 22: 24–32.

Calnan, M. (1987) *Health and Illness: The Lay Perspective*. London: Tavistock.

Cameron, P., Willis, K. and Crack, G. (1995) 'Education for Change in a Post-modern World: Redefining Revolution'. *Nurse Education Today*, 15: 336–340.

Campbell, R. and Macfarlane, A. (1987) *'Where to be born? The debate and the Evidence'*. Oxford: National Perinatal Epidemiology Unit.

Campbell, R. and Macfarlane, A. (1994) *'Where to be born? The debate and the evidence'*. (2nd edn). Oxford: National Perinatal Epidemiology Unit.

Capra, F. (1983) *The Turning Point*. New York: Bantam.

Cassell, C. and Symon, G. (1994) *Qualitative Methods in Organizational Research: A Practical Guide*. London: Sage.

Chamberlain, G., Wraight, A. and Crowley, P. (1997) Home Births. Report of the 1994 Confidential Enquiry by the National Birthday Trust Fund. Carnforth, N.Y.: Pantheon.

Chamberlain, M. (1984) 'The Making of a Male Medical Monopoly'. In A. Phillips and J. Rakusen (eds), *The New Our Bodies, Ourselves*. London: Penguin.

Chappel, E. and Coon, C. (1942) *Principles of Anthropology*. New York: Holt, Rinehart and Winston.

Charters, W.W. (1924) *Curriculum Construction*. New York: Macmillan.

Cheater, A. (1993) 'Globalization and the new technologies of knowing: anthropological calculus or chaos?' Paper presented to the Association of Social Anthropologists' Decennial Conference, St Catherine's College, Oxford, July.

Chen, P.C.Y. (1975) MD Thesis, University of Malaya, Kuala Lumpur.

Chow, R. (1992) Postmodern Automatons. In J. Butler and J. Scott (eds), *Feminist Theorize the Political*. pp. 101–117.

Clark, L., Mugford, M. and Paterson, C. (1991) 'How does the mode of delivery affect the cost of maternity care?'. *British Journal of Obstetrics and Gynaecology*, 98: 519–523.

Clarke, L. (1995) 'Nursing Research: Science, Visions and Telling Stories'. *Journal of Advanced Nursing*, 21: 584–593.

Clements, S. (1997) 'Horizontal Violence: Why Nursing Needs Radical Feminism'. *Birth Issues*, 6:(1): 9–14.

Clough, P. T. (1992) *End(s) of Ethnography: From Realism to Social Criticism*. London: Sage.

Cockerham, W.C. (1995) *The Global Society*. New York: McGraw-Hill.

Cohen, L. and Manion, L. (1994) *Research Methods in Education*. London: Routledge.

Cohen, R. (1997) *Global Diasporas: An Introduction*. London: University College London Press.

Coles, R. (1989) *The Call of Stories*. Boston, Mass.: Houghton Mifflin.

Collins, P.H. (1991) *Black Feminist Thought: Knowledge, Consciousness, and the Politics of Empowerment*. London: Harper Collins.

—— (1994) *Feminist Thought*. London: Blackwell.

Colson, A.C. (1969) PhD Thesis, Stanford University, Palo Alto.

Comaroff, J. (1977) 'Conflicting Paradigms of Pregnancy: Managing Ambiguity in Ante-Natal Encounters'. In A. Davis and G. Horobin (eds), *Medical Encounters*. London: Croom Helm.

—— (1982) 'Medicine, Symbol, and Ideology', In *The Problem of Medical Knowledge* P.P. Wright and A. Treacher, eds. Edinburgh: Edinburgh University Press.

Conrad, P. (1992) 'Medicalization and Social Control'. *Annual Review of Sociology*, 18: 209–232.

Cornia, G.A. (1999) 'Liberalisation, globalisation and income distribution'. United Nations University/WIDER Working Papers 157. Helsinki: UNU/WIDER.

Corson, D. (2000) 'Emancipatory Leadership'. *International Journal of Leadership in Education*, 3(2): 93–120.

Cosio-Zavala, M.E. and Gastineau, B. (1997) Changes in the Status of Women as a Factor and a Consequence of Changes in Family Dynamics. Report on the CICRED Seminar on Women and Families, Paris, 24–26 February.

Coulter, J. (1973) *Approaches to Insanity*. London: Martin Robertson.

Davies, D. and Neal, C. (eds) (1998) *Pink Therapy. A Guide for Counsellors Working with Lesbian, Gay and Bisexual Clients*. London: Open University Press.

Davies, I.K. (1976) *Objectives in Curriculum Design*. Maidenhead: McGraw-Hill.

Davies, J., Hey, E., Reid, W. and Young, G. (1996) Home Birth Study Steering Group. 'Prospective Regional Study of Planned Home Birth'. *British Medical Journal*, 313: 1302–1306.

Davis-Floyd, R. (1987) 'Obstetric Training as a Rite of Passage'. *Medical Anthropology Quarterly*, 1(3): 288–318.

—— (1992) *Birth as an American Rite of Passage*. Berkeley, Calif.: University of California Press.

—— (1998) 'Types of Midwifery Training: An Anthropological Overview in Pathways to Becoming a Midwife'. In J. Southern, Jennifer Rosenberg and Jan Tritten (eds), *Getting an Education*, Eugene, Oregon.

—— (2000) 'Mutual accommodation or biomedical hegemony? Anthropological perspectives on global issues in midwifery'. *Midwifery Today* 53 (Spring): 12–16, 68–69.

Davis-Floyd, R. and Davis, E. (1996) 'Intuition as Authoritative Knowledge in Midwifery and Home Birth'. In R. Davis-Floyd and Carolyn Sargent (eds), *The Social Production of Authoritative Knowledge in Childbirth. Medical Anthropology Quarterly*, (Special edn) 10(2): 237–269.

Davis-Floyd, R. and Sargent, C.F. (eds) (1997) *Childbirth and Authoritative Knowledge: Cross-Cultural Perspectives*. Berkeley, Calif.: University of California Press.

Deacon, B. and Hulse, M. (eds) (1997) *Global Social Policy*. London: Sage.

De Groot A.N.J.A., Slort, W. and Van Roosmalen J. (1993) Assessment of the Risk Approach to Maternity Care in a District Hospital in Rural Tanzania. *International Journal of Gynaecology and Obstetrics*, 40: 33–37.

Denzin, N.K. (1989) *The Research Act*. (3rd edn). New York: McGraw-Hill.

—— (1997) *Interpretive Ethnography: Ethnographic Practices for the Twenty-first Century*. London: Sage.

Denzin, N.K. and Lincoln, Y.S. (1994) *Handbook of Qualitative Research*. London: Sage.

Department of Health (1989a) *Caring for People: Community Care in the Next Decade and Beyond*. London: HMSO.

—— (1989b) *Working for Patients: Education and Training*. London: HMSO.

—— (1992) *Changing Childbirth*. Report of the Expert Maternity Group. London: HMSO.

—— (1993) *Changing Childbirth*. Report of the Expert Maternity (Cumberlege Report). London: HMSO.

—— (1996) *The Patient's Charter and Maternity Services*. London: HMSO.

—— (2002) *NHS Maternity Statistics, England: 1998–99 to 2000–01*. *http://www.doh.gov.uk/public/sb0211.htm (accessed 1.9.02)*

Department of Health and Social Security (1983) *NHS Management Inquiry Report. DHSS, Oct 25*.

Dezalay, Y. (1990) 'The Big Bang and the Law: The Internationalization and Restructuration of the Legal Field'. In M. Featherstone (ed.), *Global Culture: Nationalism, Globalization and Modernity*. London: Sage.

Doering, L. (1992) 'Power and Knowledge in Nursing: A Feminist Poststructuralist View'. *Advances in Nursing Science*, 14: 24–33.

Donnison, J. (1977) *Midwives and Medical Men*. New York: Schocken.

Douglas, M. (1966) *Purity and Danger*. London: Routledge and Kegan Paul.

Douglas, M. (1992) *Risk and Blame: Essays in Cultural Theory*. London: Routledge.

Douglas, M. (1997) 'In Defence of Shopping.' In P. Falk and C. Campbell (eds), *The Shopping Experience*. London: Sage. pp. 15–30.

Douglas, M. and Wildavsky, A. (1983) *Risk and Culture*. Berkeley, Calif.: University of California Press.

Drife, J. (1999) Data on Babies' Safety During Hospital Births are Being Ignored. *British Medical Journal*, 319(7215): 1008.

Drife, J. (1999) Maternal Mortality: Lessons from the Confidential Enquiry. *Hospital Medicine*, 60(3): 156–157.

Duffy, M.E. (1987) 'Methodological Triangulation: A Vehicle for Merging Quantitative and Qualitative Research Methods. *Image: Journal of Nursing Scholarship* 19(3): 130–133.

Dugan, S. and Dugan, D. (2000) *The Day the World Took Off – The Roots of the Industrial Revolution*. London: Channel 4 Books.

Duran, A.M. (1992) 'The Safety of Home Birth: The Farm Study'. *American Journal of Public Health*, 82(3): 450–453.

Durkheim, E. (1982) *The Rules of Sociological Method*. London: Macmillan [1895].

—— (1984) *The Division of Labour in Society*. Basingstoke: Macmillan [1895].

Ebin, V. (1982) 'Interpretations of Infertility: The Aowin People of South-west Africa'. In C.P. MacCormack (ed.), *Ethnography of Fertility and Birth*. London: Academic Press. pp. 141–160.

Ehrenreich, B. and English, D. (1973) *Witches, Midwives and Nurses: A History of Women Healers*. New York: The Feminist Press.

Eisenberg, L. (1977) 'Disease and Illness: Distinctions Between Professional and Popular Ideas of Sickness'. *Culture, Medicine and Psychiatry*, 1: 9.24.

English National Board (1988) *Evaluation of the Implementation of the Framework for Continuing Professional Education and Higher Award*. London: English National Board for Nursing, Midwifery and Health Visiting.

Enkin, M., Keirse, M.J.N.C. and Chalmers, I. (1989) *A Guide to Effective Care in Pregnancy and Childbirth*. Oxford: Oxford University Press.

Enkin, M., Keirse, M.J.N.C., Renfrew, M.J. and Neilson, J.S. (1995) *A Guide to Effective Care in Pregnancy and Childbirth*. (2nd edn). Oxford: Oxford University Press.

Enkin, M., Keirse, M.J.N.C., Renfrew, N.J. and Neilson, J.S. (2000) *A Guide to Effect-ive Care in Pregnancy and Childbirth*. (3rd edn). Oxford: Oxford University Press.

Erickson, J.A. Erikson, E., Hostlelier, J.A. and Huntington, G.E. (1979) 'Fertility Patterns and Trends Among the Old Order Amish'. *Population Studies*, 3: 255–276.

Erikson, E. (1977) 'Reflections on the American Identity'. In *Childhood and Society*. Harmondsworth: Penguin.

Escobar, A. (1988) 'Power and Visibility: Development and the Intervention and Management of the Third World'. *Cultural Anthropology*, 3(4): 428–443.

—— (1991) 'Anthropology and the Development Encounter: The Making and Marketing of Development Anthropology'. *American Ethnologist*, 18(4): 658–682.

—— (1995a) 'Power and Visibility: Tales of Peasant Women, and the Environment'. In A. Escobar (ed.), *Encountering Development: The Making and Unmaking of the Third World*. Princeton, N.J.: Princeton University Press.

Evans-Pritchard, E.E. (1972) *Witchcraft, Oracles and Magic Among the Azande*. Oxford University Press: Oxford.

Fairclough, N. (1985) 'Critical and Descriptive Goals in Discourse Analysis'. *Journal of Pragmatics*, 9: 739–763.

—— (1993) 'Critical Discourse Analysis and the Marketization of Public Discourse: The Universities'. *Discourse and Society*, 4(2): 133–168.

Fanon, F. (1967) *The Wretched of the Earth*. (trans. C. Farrington). Harmondsworth: Penguin Books.

Farrell, G. A. (1997) 'Aggression in Clinical Settings: Nurses' View'. *Journal of Advanced Nursing*, 25: 501–508.

Featherstone, M. (ed.) (1990a) *Global Culture: An Introduction Theory, Culture and Society*. pp. 1–14. London: Sage.

—— (1990b) *Global Culture: Nationalism, Globalization and Modernity*. London: Sage.

Feuerstein, M.T. (1993) *Turning the Tide. Safe Motherhood: A District Action Manual*. London: Macmillan, on behalf of Save the Children.

Field, M. (1985) 'The Jewel in the Crown: Clitoral Massage as an Analgesia for Labor'. *Childbirth Alternatives Quarterly*, 6(4): 4–5. (First published in the *Newsletter of the Association of Radical Midwives*, Winter, 1984/1985).

Figlio, Cf.K.M. (1976) 'The Metaphor of Organization: An Historiographical Per-spective on the Bio-Medical Sciences in the Early Nineteenth Century'. *History of Science*, XIV.

Fingeret, H. and Cockley, S. (1993) *'Teachers' Learning: An Evaluation of ABE Staff Development in Virginia'*. Dayton: The Virginia Adult Educators Research Network. (EDRS No. ED 356 406).

Flint, C., Pouleageris, P. and Grant, A. (1989) 'The "Know Your Midwife" Scheme: A Randomised Trial of Continuity of Care by a Team of Midwives'. Vol 22, pp. 168–169.

Fortes, M. (1950) *Kinship and Marriage*. London: Oxford University Press.

Foucault, M. (1972) *The Archaeology of Knowledge*. London: Tavistock.

Foucault, M. (1973) *The Birth of the Clinic*. London: Tavistock

—— (1977a) *Madness and Civilization: A History of Insanity in the Age of Reason*. (trans. R. Howard). London: Tavistock.

—— (1977b) *Discipline and Punishment: The Birth of the Prison*. New York: Pantheon.

—— (1980) 'Truth and Power'. In C. Gordon (ed.), *Power/Knowledges: Selected Interviews and Other Writings 1972–77*. pp. 109–133. New York: Pantheon.

—— (1984) 'The Order of Discourse'. In M. Shapiro (ed.), *Language and Politics*. New York: New York University Press. pp. 108–138.

—— (1994a) *The Birth of the Clinic. An Archaeology of Medical Perception*. New York: Vintage.

—— (1994b) *The Order of Things. An Archaeology of Human Science*. New York: Vintage.

Fraser, D. and Hammett, P. (1997) Braided Curriculum, unpublished work.

Fraser, D., Murphy, R. and Worth-Butler, M. (1997) *An Outcome of the Evaluation of the Effectiveness of Pre-Registration Midwifery Programmes of Education*. London: ENB.

Fraser, G.J. (1998) *African American Midwifery in the South: Dialogues of Birth, Race, and Memory*. Cambridge, Mass.: Harvard University Press.

Freire, P. (1972) *Pedagogy of the Oppressed*. Harmondsworth: Penguin.

Freud, S. (1938) *The Basic Writings of Sigmund Freud*. New York: Modern Library.

Friedman, J. (1989) 'The Consumption of Modernity'. *Culture and History*, 4: 117–29.

Friedman, T. (1999) *The Lexus and the Olive Tree*. London: Harper Collins.

Frosch, R.A. (1999) *The Pervasive Role of Science, Technology, and Health in Foreign Policy: Imperatives for the Department of State Office of International Affairs*. Washington: National Academies Press.

Fukuyama, F. (1996) 'Trust: Social Capital and the Global Economy'. *Current*, 379: 12.

Gadamer, H-G. (1976) Philosophical Hermeneutics. (trans. and ed. D.E. Lingo). Berkeley, Calif.: University of California Press.

Garcia, J., Kilpatrick, R. and Richards, M. (1990) *The Politics of Maternity Care: Services for Childbearing Women in Twentieth-Century Britain*. Oxford: Clarendon.

Gaskin, I.M. (1990) *Spiritual Midwifery* (3rd edn). Summertown, Team.: Book Pub. Co.

Gessner, V. and Schade, A. (1990) 'Conflicts of Culture in Cross-Border Legal Relations: The Conception of a Research Topic in the Sociology of Law'. In M. Featherstone (ed.), *Global Culture: Nationalism, Globalization and Modernity*. London: Sage.

Ghana Statistical Service (1998) Ghana Demographic and Health Surveys. Ghana Statistical Service.

Gibson, F. (1999) Science, Midwifery Politics and the Clinical Characteristics of the Midwifery Model of Care – more than just 'non-intervention'. Information for Obstetricians. GoodNewsNetwork. *http://www.domiciliary.org/acdm-va/obinfo.html*

Giddens, A. (1989) *Sociology*. Cambridge: Polity.

—— (1990) *The Consequences of Modernity*. Cambridge: Polity.

—— (1991) *Modernity and Self Identity: Self and Society in the Late Modern Age*. Cambridge: Polity.

—— (1997) *Sociology*. (3rd edn). Cambridge, Polity.

Gifford, D. (1990) *The Farther Shore: A Natural History of Perception 1798–1984*. London: Faber and Faber.

Ginsburg, F.D. and Rapp, R. (eds) (1995) *Conceiving the New World Order: The Global Politics of Reproduction*. Berkeley, Calif.: University of California Press.

Glennon, L.M. (1979) *Women and Dualism: A Sociology of Knowledge Analysis*. New York: Longman.

Goer, H. (1995) *Obstetric Myths Versus Research Realities: A Guide to the Medical Literature*. Westport, Conn.: Bergin & Garvey.

Goffman, E. (1961) *Asylums: Essay on the Social Situation of Mental Patients and Other Inmates*. Harmondsworth: Penguin.

Gordon, G. (1990) *Training Manual for Traditional Birth Attendants*. London: Macmillan.

Goss, J.D. and Leinbach, T.R. (1996) 'Focus Groups as Alternative Research Practice'. *Area*, 28 (2): 115–23.

Gramsci, A. (1971) *Selections from the Prison Notebooks of Antonio Gramsci* (ed. and trans. by Q. Hoare and G. Nowell-Smith). London: Lawrence and Wishart.

Gribble, J.H. (1970) 'Pandora's Box: The Affective Domain of Educational Objectives'. *Journal of Curriculum Studies*, 2(1):11–24.

Guess, R. (1981) *The Idea of a Critical Theory: Habermas and the Frankfurt School*. Cambridge: Cambridge University Press.

Guillemette, J. and Fraser, W.D. (1992) 'Differences Between Obstetricians in Caesarean Section Rates and the Management of Labour'. *British Journal of Obstetrics and Gynaecology*, 99: 105–108.

Habermas, J. (1971) *Towards a Rational Society*. London: Heinemann.

—— (1978) *The Critical Theory of Jurgen Habermas*. (edited by T. McCarthy). Cambridge, Mass.: MIT Press.

Habermas, J. (1978) *Knowledge and Human Interests*. (trans. J.J. Shapuro). London: Heinemannn.

Hall, S. (1992) 'The Question of Cultural Identity'. In S. Hall *et al.* (eds), *Modernity and its Futures*. Cambridge: Polity and Open University Press. pp. 273–316.

Hamelink, C. (1983) *Cultural Autonomy in Global Communications*. New York: Longman.

Hammersley, M. and Atkinson, P. (1983) *Ethnography: Principles in Practice*. London: Tavistock.

Handlin, O. (1972) 'Ambivalence in the Popular Response to Science'. In B. Barnes (ed.), *Sociology of Science*. Harmondsworth: Penguin.

Hannerz, U. (1989) 'Culture Between Center and Periphery: Toward a Macroanthropology'. *Ethnos*, 54: 200–216.

—— (1990) 'Cosmopolitan and Locals in World Cultures'. In M. Featherstone (ed.), *Global Culture: Nationalism, Globalization and Modernity*. London: Sage. pp. 237–251.

—— (1992) *Cultural Complexity: Studies in the Social Organisation of Meaning*. New York: Columbia University Press.

—— (1996) *Transnational Connections: Culture, People, Places*. London: Routledge.

Harding, S. (1987) *Feminism and Methodology*. Bloomington and Indianapolis: Indiana University Press.

—— (1991) *Whose Science? Whose Knowledge?: Thinking from Women's Lives*. Milton Keynes: Open University Press.

Harper, D. (1987) *Working Knowledge*. Chicago: Chicago University Press.

Harraway, D. (1991) *Simians, Cyborgs, and Women: The Reinvention of Nature*. London: Free Association Books.

Hartman, B. (1987) *Reproductive Rights and Wrongs. The Global Politics of Population Control and Contraceptive Choice*. New York: Harper & Row.
—— (1995) *Reproductive Rights and Wrongs and the Global Politics of Population Control*. Cambridge, Mass.: South End Press.
Harvey, D. (1989) *The Condition of Postmodernity*. Oxford: Blackwell.
—— (1992) *The Condition of Postmodernity. An Enquiry into the Origins of Cultural Change*. Cambridge, MA: Blackwell.
Hastie, C. (1995) 'Midwives Eat Their Young Don't They?' *Birth Issues*, 4: 5–9.
Hawley, A. (1981) *Urban Society: An Ecological Approach*. New York: John Wiley.
Heap, S.H. and Ross, A. (1992) *Understanding the Enterprise Culture: Themes in the Work of Mary Douglas*. Edinburgh: Edinburgh University Press.
Hedin, B. (1986) 'A Case Study of Oppressed Group Behaviour in Nurses'. *Image: Journal of Nursing Scholarship*, 18(2): 53–57.
Henderson, C. and Jones, K. (1997) *Essential Midwifery*. London: Mosby.
Hewitt, T. (2000) 'A consideration of the usefulness of computer-based technology as a means by which people with learning disabilities might exert some influence on the decision-making processes that affect the services that they use'. Unpublished Masters Paper. Anglia Polytechnic University.
Hobbes, T. (1998) *Leviathan* [1651] (edited by J.C.A. Gaskin). Oxford: Oxford World Classics.
Hodges, S. (1996) 'Midwifery Model of Care'. *Citizens for Midwifery News*, 1(1)
Hofstede, G. (1991) *Cultures and Organizations: Software of the Mind*. London: McGraw-Hill.
Honeycutt, L. (1994) What Hath Bakhtin Wrought: Toward a Unified Theory of Literature and Composition. Master's thesis, UNC Charlotte.
   http://www.public.iastate.edu/~honeyl/bakhtin/thesis.html
Horton, R. (1971) 'African Traditional Thought and Western Science'. In M.F.D. Young (ed.), *Knowledge and Control: New Directions in the Sociology of Education*. London: Collier-Macmillan. pp. 208–265.
Humphrey, M., Chang, A., Wood, E.L., Morgan, S. and Hounslow, D. (1974) 'The Decrease in Fetal pH During the Second Stage of Labour when Conducted in the Dorsal Position'. *Journal of Obstetric Gynaecology, British Commonwealth*, 81: 600–602.
Humphrey, M., Hounslow, D., Morgan, S. and Wood, C. (1973) 'The Influence of Maternal Posture at Birth of Fetus'. *Journal of Obstetric Gynaecology, British Commonwealth*, 80: 1075–80
Hundley, V.A., Cruickshank, F.M. and Lang, G.D. (1994) 'Midwife Managed Delivery Unit: A Randomised Controlled Comparison with Consultant-led Care'. *British Medical Journal*, 309: 1400–1404.
Hunter, B. (1999) 'Oral History and Research part 1: Uses and Implications'. *British Journal of Midwifery*, (7)7: 426–429.
—— (1999) 'Oral History and Research part 2: Current Practice'. *British Journal of Midwifery*, (7)8: 481–484.
Idarius, B. (1999) 'The Midwifery Model of Care'. *Sojourn Magazine*, 3(3).
   http://www.sojourn.org/sojourn/summer99/default.html
Illich, I. (1976) *Limits of Medicine – Medical Nemesis: The Exploration of Health*. London: Boyars.
—— (1977) *Disabling Professions*. London: Boyars.

Jackson, N.V. and Irvine, L.M. (1998) 'The Influence of Maternal Requests on the Elective Caesarean Section Rate'. *Journal of Obstetrics and Gynaecology*, 18: 115–119.

Jacobus, M., Fox Keller, E. and Shuttleworth, S. (eds) (1990) *Body/Politics: Women and the Discourse of Science*. New York: Routledge.

Jarvis, P. (1992) *Paradoxes of Learning*. San Francisco, Calif.: Jossey Bass.

—— (1999) *The Practitioner-Researcher: Developing Theory from Practice*. San Francisco, Calif.: Jossey-Bass.

—— (2000) 'The Practitioner-Researcher in Nursing'. *Journal of Advanced Nursing*, 20(1): 30–35.

Jick, T. (1993) 'Mixing Qualitative and Quantitative Methods: Triangulation in Action'. In J. Van Maanen (ed.), *Qualitative Methodology*. Newbury Park, Calif.: Sage. pp. 135–148.

Jomo, Kwame Sundaram (1988) *A Question of Class: Capital, the State, and Uneven Development in Malaya*. New York: Monthly Review Press.

Jordan, B. (1983) *Birth in Four Cultures: A Cross-Cultural Investigation of Childbirth in Yucatan, Holland, Sweden and the United States*. Montreal: Eden Press.

—— (1993) *Birth in Four Cultures: A Cross-Cultural Investigation of Childbirth in Yucatan, Holland, Sweden and the United States*. (4th edn). Prospect Heights, Ill.: Waveland Press.

Jordan, B. and Irwin, S. (1989) 'The Ultimate Failure: Court-Ordered Cesarean Section'. In L. Whiteford and M. Poland (eds), *New Approaches to Human Reproduction*. Boulder, Colo.: Westview Press. pp. 13–24.

Justice, J. (1984) 'Can Socio-Cultural Information Improve Health Planning? A Case Study of Nepal's Assistant Nurse Midwife.' *Social Science and Medicine*, 19(3): 193–198.

—— (1986) *Policies, Plans, and People: Foreign Aid and Health Development*. Berkeley, Calif.: University of California Press.

—— (1986) 'The Bureaucratic Context of International Health: A Social Scientist's View'. *Social Science and Medicine*, 25: 1301–1306.

Kawachi, I., Kennedy, B.P. and Lochner, K. (1997) 'Long Live Community: Social Capital As Public Health'. *The American Prospect*, 35. 56.

Kearl, M.C. (1989) *Endings: A Sociology of the Dying and the Dead*. New York: Dolphin Books.

Keddie, N. (1980) 'Ideology of Individualism'. In J.L.Thompson (ed.), *Adult Education for a Change*. London: Hutchinson.

Kelly, A.V. (1989) *The Curriculum: Theory and Practice*. (3rd edn). London: Paul Chapman.

King, A. (1990) *Global Cities*. London: Routledge.

—— (1990) 'Architecture, Capital and the Globalization of Culture'. In M. Featherstone (ed.), *Global Culture: Nationalism, Globalization and Modernity*. London: Sage.

Kirkham, M.J. and Perkins, E.R. (1997) *Reflections on Midwifery*. London: Ballière Tindall.

Kitzinger J. (1994) 'The Methodology of Focus Groups: the Importance of Interaction Between Research Participants'. *Sociology of Health*, 16(1): 103–121.

Kitzinger J. (1995) 'Introducing Focus Groups'. *British Medical Journal*, 311: 299–302.

Kitzinger, S. (1972) *The Experience of Childbirth*. (3rd edn). Harmondsworth: Penguin.

Kliewer, J.R. (1999) *The Innovative Campus: Nurturing the Distinctive Learning Environment*. Phoenix: Oryx Press.

Kloos, P. (1999) 'The Dialectics of Globalization and Localization'. In D. Kalb, M. van der Land, R. Staring and B. van Steenbergen (eds), *Globalization, Inequality and Difference. Consequences of Transnational Flows*. Oxford: Rowman & Littlefield. *http://casnws.scw.vu.nl/publicaties/kloos-dialectics.html*

Korten, D. (1995) *When Corporations Rule the World*. West Hartford, Conn:. Kumarian Press.

Kreuger R.A. (1988) *Focus Groups: A Practical Guide for Applied Research*. London: Sage.

Lankshear A.J. (1993) 'The Use of Focus Groups in a Study of Attitudes to Student Nurse Assessment'. *Journal of Advanced Nursing*, 18: 1986–89.

Lash, S. and Urry, J. (1994) *Economies of Signs and Space*. London: Sage.

Laslett, P. (1999) *The World We Have Lost*. London: Routledge.

Lave, J. and Wenger, E. (1991) *Situated Learning: Legitimate Peripheral Participation*. Cambridge: Cambridge University Press.

Lawton, D. (1973) *The New Social Studies: Handbook for Teachers in Primary, Secondary and Further Education*. London: Heinemann.

Lay, M.M. (2000) *The Rhetoric of Midwifery: Gender, Knowledge, and Power*. New Jersey: Rutgers University Press.

Layder, D. (1997) *Modern Social Theory: Key Debates and New Directions*. London: University of Leicester Press.

Leap, N. (1997) 'Making sense of "horizontal violence" in midwifery'. *British Journal of Midwifery*, 5(11): 689.

Leap, N. and Hunter, B. (1993) *The Midwife's Tale: An Oral History from Handywoman to Professional Midwife*. London: Scarlet Press.

LeCompte, M.D. (1993) 'A Framework for Hearing Silence: What Does Telling Stories Mean When We Are Supposed to be Doing Science?' In D. McLaughlin and W.G. Tierney (eds), *Naming Silenced Lives: Personal Narratives and Processes of Educational Change*. London: Routledge. pp. 9–27.

Leitch, V.B. (1996) *Postmodernism – Local Effects, Global Flows*. Albany, N.Y.: Suny Press.

Levitt, Marta (1987) 'A Systematic Study of Birth and Traditional Birth Attendants in Nepal'. Kathmandu: John Snow Inc.

Levitt, R., Wall, A. and Appleby, J. (1999) *The Reorganised National Health Service*. London: Nelson Thornes.

Levy, M. (1966) *Modernization and the Structure of Societies*. Princeton: Princeton University Press.

Lewis, O. (1966) 'The Culture of Poverty'. *Scientific America*, 215(4): 19–25.

Lim, M.H. (1982) 'Capitalism and Industrialization in Malaysia'. *Bulletin of Concerned Asian Scholars*, 14(1): 32–47.

Litoff, J.B. (1978) *American Midwives*. Westport: Greenwood.

Litsios, S. (1997) Analysis of National Reports on the Third Evaluation of the Strategy for Health For All.

Lowndes, V. (2000) 'Women and Social Capital: A Comment on Hall's "Social Capital in Britain"'. *British Journal of Political Science*, 30(3): 533.

Lubic, R. (1994) 'Barriers and Conflicts in Maternity Care Innovation'. Conference proceedings, *Birth Issues – Choice, Control and Decision Making*. CAPERS, 1994.

Lyotard, J-F. (1984) *The Postmodern Condition: A Report on Knowledge*. Manchester: Manchester University Press.

Lytle, S.L., Belzer, A. and Reumann, R. (1993) *Initiating Practitioner Inquiry: Adult Literacy Teachers, Tutors, and Administrators Research Their Practice*. (Technical Report TR93–11). Philadelphia, Pa.: National Center on Adult Literacy.

MacIntosh J. (1981) 'Focus Groups in Distance Nursing Education'. *Journal of Advanced Nursing*, 18: 1981–85.

MacIntyre, A.C. (1964) 'Against Utilitarianism'. In T.H.B. Hollins (ed.), *Aims in Education: The Philosophic Approach*. Manchester: Manchester University Press.

Maclean, G.D. (1998) A Examination of the Characteristics of Short Term Midwifery International Consultants. PhD Thesis, University of Surrey, Guildford.

McAllister, C. (1987) Matriliny, Islam and Capitalism: Combined and Uneven Development in the Lives of the Negeri Sembilan Women. Doctoral Dissertation, University of Pittsburgh. pp. 88–93.

—— (1989a) 'Putting on the Veil: Islamic Revival as Women's Response to Development in Negeri Sembilan, Malaysia'. Paper presented at the National Women's Studies Association Annual Conference, Towson, Md.

—— (1989b) 'Padi Fields, Rubber Trees, and Education: Reconstructions of Matriliny and Gender in Negeri Sembilan, Malaysia'. Paper presented at the American Anthropological Association Annual Meetings, Washington, D.C.

—— (1992) ' "It's Our Adat": Capitalist Development and the Revival of Tradition among women in Negeri Sembilan, Malaysia'. In Patricia Lyons Johnson (ed.), *Balancing Acts: Women and the Process of Social Change*. Boulder, Colo.: Westview Press.

McCall, E. (1996) 'Horizontal Violence in Nursing: The Continuing Silence'. *The Lamp*, April: 28–30.

McConkey, D. and Lawler, P.A. (eds) (2000) *Social Structures, Social Capital, and Personal Freedom*. Westport, Conn.: Praeger.

McCormack, C. (1994) 'The Health Promotion Gap'. *Healthlines*, 13: 10.

McGurgan, P., Coulter-Smith, S. and O'Donnovan, P.J. (2001) 'A National Confidential Survey of Obstetrician's Personal Preferences Regarding Mode of Delivery'. *European Journal of Obstetrics and Gynecology and Reproductive Biology*, 97: 17–19.

McKay, S. and Mahan, C. (1984) 'Laboring Patients Need More Freedom to Move'. *Contemporary Obstetrics and Gynecology* July, 119.

—— (1988) 'Modifying the stomach contents of laboring women: why and how; successes and risks'. *Birth*, 15(4): 213–21.

McKeown, T. (1965) *Medicine in Modern Society*. London: George Allen & Unwin.

—— (1976) *The Modern Rise of Population*. New York: Academic.

McLaren, P. (1992) 'Collisions with Otherness: "Travelling" Theory, Post-Colonial Criticism, and the Politics of Ethnographic Practice – the Mission of the Wounded Ethnographer'. *Qualitative Studies in Education*, 5(1): 77–92.

McLuhan, M. (1962) 'The New Electronic Interdependence Recreates the World in the Image of a Global Village'. In *The Gutenberg Galaxy*. London: Routledge and Kegan Paul.

—— (1964) *Understanding Media*. London: Routledge.

McLuhan, M., Fiore, Q. and Angel, J. (1968) *War and Peace in the Global Village*. New York: Bantam.

Mager, R.F. (1962) *Preparing Instructional Objectives*. Palo Alto, Calif.: Fearson.

Maglacas, A.M. and Simons, J. (eds) (1986) *The Potential of the Traditional Birth Attendant*. Geneva: World Health Organization.

Mahler, H. (1987) 'The Safe Motherhood Initiative: A Call to Action'. *Lancet* 1(8534): 668–70.

Mandel, E. (1980) *Late Capitalism*. London: New Left Books.

Mannheim, K. (1960) *Ideology and Utopia: An introduction to the Sociology of Knowledge*. London: Routledge and Kegan Paul.

Marcuse, H. (1972) *One Dimensional Man*. London, Abacus.

Marland, H. and Rafferty, A.M. (1997) *Midwives, Society and Childbirth: Debates and Controversies in the Modern Period*. London: Routledge.

Marshall, P. (ed.) (1997) *The Impact of the English Reformation 1500–1640*. London: Arnold.

Martin, E. (1987) *The Woman in the Body*. Boston: Beacon Press.

Martin-Prevel, Y., Delpeuch, F., Traissac, P., Massambam, J-P., Aduoa-Oyila, G., Coudert, K. and Trèche, S. (2000) 'Deterioration in the Nutritional Status of Young Children and Their Mothers in Brazzaville, Congo, Following the 1994 Devaluation of the CFA Franc'. *World Health Bulletin*, 78: 108–118.

Marx, K. (1970) *Capital*, vol 1. London: Lawrence and Wishart [1864].

Mass, B. (1976) *Population Target: The Political Economy of Population Control in Latin America*. Toronto: Women's Press.

Maternal and Child Health Research Consortium (1998) 'Confidential Enquiry into Stillbirths and Deaths in Infancy'. Fifth Annual Report. London: Maternal and Child Health Research Consortium, pp. 51–62.

Mead, M. and Newton, N. (1967) 'Cultural Patterning of Perinatal Behaviour'. In S.A. Richardson and A.F. Guttmacher (eds), *Childbearing: Its Social and Psychological Aspects*. Baltimore, Md.: Williams and Wilkins.

Mehl, L.E., Pererson, G.H., Whitt, M. and Hawes, W.H. (1977a) 'Outcomes of Elective Home Births: A Series of 1,146 Cases'. *Journal of Reproductive Medicine*, 19(5): 281–290.

—— (1977b) 'Research on Childbirth Alternatives: What Can it tell Us About Hospital practice? In D. Stewart and L. Stewart (eds), *21st Century Obstetrics Now!* Marble Hill, Mo.: NAPSAC (International Association of Parents and Professionals for Safe Alternatives in Childbirth).

Mehmet, O. (1995) *Westernizing the Third World. The Eurocentricity of Economic Development Theory*. London: Routledge.

Merchant, C. (1983) *The Death of Nature: Women, Ecology, and the Scientific Revolution*. San Francisco, Calif.: Harper and Row.

Merton, T. (1968) 'Puritanism, Pietism and Science'. In J.K. Merton (ed.), *Social Theory and Social Structure*. New York: Free Press; London: Collier-Macmillan. pp. 628–649.

Mezirow, J. (1990) 'How Critical Reflection Triggers Transformative Learning'. In J. Mezirow and Associates (eds), *Fostering Critical Reflection in Adulthood: A Guide to Transformative and Emancipatory Learning*. San Francisco, Calif.: Jossey-Bass.

Mill, J.S. (1991) *Liberty, Equality, Fraternity* [1873]. Chicago: University of Chicago Press.

Miller, D. (1997) *Capitalism: An Ethnographic Approach (Explorations in Anthropology)*. Oxford: Berg.

Miller, T. (1998) 'Shifting Layers of Professional, Lay and Personal Narratives: Longitudinal Childbirth Research'. In J. Ribbens and R. Edwards (eds), *Feminist Dilemmas in Qualitative Research: Public Knowledge and Private Lives*. London: Sage. pp. 58–71.

Millette, B. (1993) 'Client Advocacy and the Moral Orientation of Nurses'. *Western Journal of Nursing Research*, 15 (5): 607–618.

Milner, A. (1994) *Contemporary Cultural Theory*. London: UCL Press.

Miner, H. (1975) 'Body Ritual among the Nacirema'. In J.P. Spradley, and M.A. Rynkiewich (eds), *The Nacirema: Readings on American Culture*. Boston, Mass.: Little, Brown. Cited in R. Davis-Floyd (1992) *Birth as an American Rite of Passage*. Berkeley, Calif.: University of California Press.

Ministry of Health Malaysia (1990) Midwifery Curriculum (One Year).

Mitchell, E.S. (1986) 'Multiple Triangulation: A Methodology for Nursing Science'. *Advances in Nursing Science*, 8 (3): 18–26.

Mitler, L.K., Rizzo, J.A. and Horwitz, S.M. (2000) Physician Gender and Cesarean Sections. *Journal of Clinical Epidemiology*, 53:1030–1035.

Moghaddam, F.M. (1997) *The Specialized Society: The Plight of the Individual in an Age of Individualism*. Westport, Conn.; London: Praeger.

Moore, S.F. and Myerhoff, B. (eds) (1977) *Secular Ritual*. Assen, The Netherlands: Van Gorcum.

Morgan, D.L. (1997) *Focus Groups as Qualitative Research*. (2nd edn). London: Sage.

Morgan, D.L. and Spanish, M.T. (1984) 'Focus Groups: A New Tool for Qualitative Research'. *Qualitative Sociology*, 7: 253–270.

Morgan, G. (1997) *Images of Organizations*. London: Sage.

Morsy, S.A. and El-Bayoumi, J. (1993) 'Risk as an Analytical Construct: Implications for Children's Health in Arab societies'. *Childhood*, 1(2): 63–75.

Mugford, M. (1990) 'Economies of Scale and Low Risk Maternity Care: What is the Evidence?' *Maternity Action*, 46: 6–8. (newsletter of Maternity Alliance).

—— (1993) 'The Costs of Continuous Electronic Fetal Monitoring in Low Risk Labour'. In J.A.D. Spencer and R.H.T. Ward (eds), *Intrapartum Fetal Surveillance*. London: RCOG Press. pp. 241–252.

Navarro, V. (1976) *Medicine under Capitalism*. New York: Prodist.

—— (1986) *Crisis, Health and Medicine: A Social Critique*. New York: Tavistock.

Negussie, B. (1990) 'Mother and Child Care, Child Development and Child-Rearing in East African Perspective'. Paper produced for the Consultative Group on Early Childhood Care and Development.

Nelson, L.H. (1993) 'Epistemological Communities'. In L. Alcoff and E. Potter (eds), *Feminist Epistemologies*. London: Routledge.

Nelson, M.K. (1983) 'Working-Class Women, Middle-Class Women and Models of Childbirth'. *Social Problems*, 30(3): 284–297.

Nelson, N. and Wright, S. (1995) *Power and Participatory Development*. London: Intermediate Technology.

Newton, N. (1973) 'The Interrelationship between Sexual Responsiveness, Birth and Breastfeeding'. In J. Zubin and J. Moore (eds), *Contemporary Sexual Behavior: Critical Issues in the 1970s*. Baltimore, Md.: New York: Johns Hopkins University Press.

—— (1977) *Maternal Emotions: A Study of Women's Feelings toward Menstruation, Pregnancy, Childbirth, Breastfeeding, Infant Care and Other Aspects of Femininity*. Paul B. Hoeber.

Nolan, M. and Behi, R. (1995) 'Triangulation: The Best of all Worlds?' *British Journal of Nursing*, 4: 829–832.

Northern Region Perinatal Mortality Survey Coordinating Group (1996) Collaborative Survey of Perinatal Loss in Planned and Unplanned Home Births. *British Medical Journal*, 313: 1306–1309.

Oakley, A. (1975) 'The Trap of Medicalized Motherhood'. *New Society* 34, 689: 639–641.

—— (1991) 'Using Medical Care: The Views and Experiences of High-Risk Mothers'. *Health Services Research*, 26(5): 651–669.

—— (1992) *Social Support and Motherhood*. Oxford: Blackwell.

—— (1993) *Essays on Women and Health*. Edinburgh: Edinburgh University Press.

—— (2000) *Experiments in Knowing: Gender and the Method of Social Sciences*. Cambridge: Polity.

Oakley, A. and Houd, S. (eds) (1990) *Helpers in Childbirth: Midwifery Today*. New York; London: Hemisphere Publishing Corporation.

Odent, M. (1984) *Birth Reborn*. New York: Pantheon.

OECD (Organization for Economic Co-operation and Development) (1993) Special Issue on Globalization, STI Review 13.

Office for National Statistics (2000) Child Health Statistics. (2nd edn). London: The Stationery Office.

Office for National Statistics (2002) *Health Statistics Quarterly*, 13, Spring 2002.

Ong, A. (1983) *Global Industries and Malay Peasants in West Malaysia*. In June Nash and Maria Patricia Fernadez-Kelly (eds), *Women, Men and the International Division of Labor*. Albany, N.Y.: State University of New York Press. pp. 426–439.

—— (1987) *Spirit of Resistance and Capitalist Discipline: Factory Women in Malaysia*. Albany, NY.: State University of New York Press.

Oppong, C. and Abu, K. (1987) *Seven Roles of Women: Impact of Education, Migration and Employment of Ghanaian Mothers*. International Labour Office.

Orwell, G. Quoted in Wade, N. (1974) 'Bottle Feeding: Adverse Effects of Western Technology'. *Science*, 184: 45–48.

Osterman, K.F. and Kottkamp, R.B. (1993) *Reflective Practice for Educators: Improving Schooling Through Professional Development*. Newbury Park, Calif.: Corwin Press.

Oxorn, H. and Foote, W.R. (1975) *Human Labor and Birth*. (3rd edn). New York: Appleton-Century-Crofts.

Pansini-Murrell, J. (1996) 'Incorporating Problem-based Learning: Striving towards Women-Centred Care'. *British Journal of Midwifery*, 4(9): 479–482.

Parker, J. and Gardner, G. (1992) 'The Silence and the Silencing of the Nurses' Voice'. *Australian Journal of Advanced Nursing*, 9(2): 3–9.

Parkin, D. (1993) 'Nemi in the Modern World: Return of the Exotic'. *Man*, 28: 79–99.

Parsons, T. (1951) *The Social System*. London: Routledge and Kegan Paul.

—— (1964) 'Evolutionary Universals in Society'. *American Sociological Review*, 29: 339–357.

—— (1964) *Social Structure and Personality*. London: Collier-Macmillan.

—— (1977) *The Evolution of Societies*. Englewood Cliffs: Prentice-Hall.

Pavis, S., Masters, H. and Cunningham-Burley, S. (eds) (1996) Lay Concepts of Positive Mental Health and How it can be Maintained. Final Report to Health Education Board for Scotland.

Pedler, M., Burgoyne, J. and Boydell, T. (1991) *The Learning Company: A Strategy for Sustainable Development*. London: McGraw Hill.

Pigg, Stacy Leigh (1991) 'Unintended Consequences: The Ideological Impact of Development in Nepal'. *South Asia Bulletin*, 8(1–2): 45–58.

—— (1992) 'Inventing Social Categories Through Place: Social Representations and Development in Nepal'. *Comparative Studies in Society and History*, 34(3): 491–513.

—— (1995a) 'The Credible and the Credulous: The Question of "Villagers' Beliefs" in Nepal'. *Cultural Anthropology*, 11(2): 160–201.

—— (1995b) 'Acronyms and Effacement: Traditional Medical Practitioners (TMP) in International Health Development'. *Social Science and Medicine*, 41(1) (1995): 47–68.

Poirier, S. and Ayres, L. (1997) Focus on Qualitative Methods – Endings, Secrets, and Silences: Overreading in Narrative Inquiry. *Research in Nursing and Health*, 20: 551–557.

Polanyi, M. (1967) *The Tacit Dimension*. London: Routledge and Kegan Paul.

Poma, P.A. (1999) 'Effects of Obstetrician Characteristics on Cesarean Delivery Rates: A Community Hospital Experience'. *American Journal of Obstetrics and Gynecology*, 180: 1354–72.

Population Crisis Committee (1988) 'Country Rankings of the Status of Women: poor, Powerless and Pregnant'. *Population, Briefing Paper* 20 (June): 5.

Porter, T. (1995) *Trust in Numbers: the Pursuit of Objectivity in Science and Public Life*. Princeton N.J.: Princeton University Press.

Portes, A. (2000) 'The Two Meanings of Social Capital'. *Sociological Forum*, 15(1): 1.

Powell, R.A. and Single, H.M. (1996) 'Focus groups'. *International Journal of Quality in Health Care*, 8(5): 499–504.

Powell, R.A., Single H.M. and Lloyd, K.R. (1996) 'Focus Groups in Mental Health Research: Enhancing the Validity of User and Provider Questionnaires'. *International Journal of Social Psychology*, 42(3): 193–206.

Powles, J. (1971) 'On the Limitations of Modern Medicine'. *Science, Medicine and Man*, 1: 1–30.

Pritchard, J.A. and MacDonald, P.C. (1980) *Williams Obstetrics*. (16th edn). New York: Appleton-Century-Crofts.

Priya, Dr. J.V. (1992) *Birth Traditions: Modern Pregnancy Care*. Shaftesbury: Element.

Prosono, M. (1993) *Professional Dominance and History: Commissions of Lunacy and their Impact on the Institutionalization of Medical Authority*. Springfield, Mo.: M. Prosono.

Punnet, L. (1990) 'The Politics of Menstrual Extraction'. In Marlene Gerber Fried (ed.) *From Abortion to Reproductive Freedom: Transforming a Movement*. Boston, South End Press.

—— (1995) 'Acronyms and Effacement: Traditional Medical Practitioners (TMP) in International Health Development'. *Social Science and Medicine*, 41(1) (1995): 47–68.

Putnam, R.D. (2001) *Bowling Alone: The Collapse and Revival of American Community*. New York: Touchstone.

Putnam, R.D., Leonardi, R. and Nanatti, R.Y. (1993) *Making Democracy Work: Civic Traditions in Modern Italy*. Princeton, N.J.: Princeton University Press.

Race K.E., Hotch D.F. and Parker T. (1994) 'Rehabilitation Program Evaluation: Use of Focus Groups to Empower Clients'. *Evaluation Review* 18(6): 730–40.

Rattray, R.S. (1923) *Ashanti*. London: Oxford University Press.

—— (1969) *Tribes of the Ashanti Hinterland*. Oxford: Oxford University Press.

Read, G.D. (1972) *Childbirth Without Fear*. (4th edn). revised by Helen Wessel and Harlan F. Ellis MD). New York: Harper & Row.

Reason, P. and Rowan, J. (1991) Human Inquiry. (7th edn). London: John Wiley and Sons.

Register of Best Practices on Indigenous Knowledge (2000)
   http://www.unesco.org/most/bpikreg.htm

Reich, R.B. (1991) *The World of Nations*. New York: Knopf.

Reynolds, R.F. (1983) 'Churching of Women'. In J.R. Strayer (ed.), *Dictionary of the Middle Ages*, vol 3. New York: Charles Scribner.

Riegel, K.F. (1978) *Psychology Mon Amour: A Countertext*. Boston: Houghton Mifflin.

Roberts, J. (1986) 'Games Nurses Play'. *American Journal of Nursing*, July: 848–849.

Roberts, S. (1994) 'Oppressed Group Behaviour: Implications for Nursing'. *Revolution, the Journal of Nurse Empowerment*, Fall: 29–35.

Robertson, R. (1987) Globalization Theory and Civilizational Analysis. *Comparative Civilizations Review*, 17: 20–30.

—— (1990) 'Mapping the Global Condition: Globalization as the Central Concept'. In M. Featherstone (ed.), *Global Culture: Nationalism, Globalization and Modernity*. London: Sage.

—— (1992) *Globalization: Social Theory and Global Culture*. London: Sage.

—— (1994) 'Globalization or Glocalization'. *Journal of International Communication*, 1: 33–52.

Roger, C. (1983) *Freedom to Learn*. London: Merrill.

Romalis, S. (1981) *Taking Care of the Little Woman. Childbirth: Alternatives to Medical Control*. Austin, Tex.: University of Texas Press.

Romanyshyn, R.D. and Whalen, B.J. (1987) 'Depression and the American Dream. The Struggle with Home'. In D.M. Levin (ed.), *Pathologies of the Modern Self. Postmodern Studies in Narcissism, Schizophrenia, and Depression*. New York: New York University Press, pp. 198–220.

Rooney C. (1992) *Antenatal Care and Maternal Health: How effective is it? A Review of the Evidence*. Geneva: World Health Organization.

Rosaldo, M.Z. and Lamphere, L. (1974) *Woman, Culture and Society*. Palo Alto, Calif.: Stanford University Press.

Rosen, M.G. and Dickinson, J.C. (1993) 'The paradox of electronic fetal monitoring: more data may not enable us to predict or prevent infant neurologic morbidity'. *Am J Obstet Gynecol*, 168(3 Part I): 745–51.

Rosenfield, A. and Maine, D. (1985) 'Maternal Mortality – A Neglected Tragedy: Where is the M in MCH?' *Lancet*, 2: 83–85.

Rothman, B.K. (1990) Midwives in Transition: The Structure of a Clinical Revolution. In P. Conrad and R. Kern (eds), *The Sociology of Health and Illness Critical Perspectives*. (3rd edn). New York: St. Martin's Press.

Rowson, M. (2002) Equity and Global Economic and Health Policies: A Northern

NGO Perspective. In A. Oliver (ed.), *International Perspectives on Equity and Health*: As Seen from the UK. *Proceedings from a meeting of the Health Equity Network*. The Nuffield Trust, London.

Sandall, J. (1995) 'Choice, Continuity and Control: Changing Midwifery, Towards a Sociological Perspective'. *Midwifery*, 11: 201–209.

Savage, W. (1986) *A Savage Enquiry: Who Controls Childbirth?* London: Virago.

Schan, P. (1998) 'Lost in a Maze'. *Midwifery Matters*, 77 Summer.

Schlenzka, P.F. (1999) Safety of alternative approaches to childbirth. Unpublished dissertation, Stanford University Press.

Schon, D. (1988) 'From Technical Rationality to Reflection-in-Action'. In J. Dowie and A. Elstein (eds), *Professional Judgement*. Milton Keynes: Open University Press.

Schuller, T. and Bamford, C. (2000) 'A Social Capital Approach to the Analysis of Continuing Education: Evidence from a UK Learning Society Research Programme'. *Oxford Review of Education*, 26(1): 5.

Schwarz, M. and Thompson, M. (1990) *Divided We Stand: Redefining, Politics Technology and Social Choice*. Hemel Hempstead: Harvester-Wheatsheaf.

Scott, M. (1989) 'Brave New World: The Lives of Malaysian, especially Malay, Women Transformed by Factory Work'. *Far Eastern Economic Review*, December 21.

Scully, D. (1981) *Men who Control Women's Health: The Miseducation of Obstetrician-gynecologists*. Boston, Mass.: Houghton-Mifflin.

Shapiro, T. M. (1985) *Population Control: Women, Sterilization, and Reproductive Choice*. Philadelphia, Pa.: Temple University Press.

Sharp, J. and Hobby, E. (1999) *The Midwives Book: Or the Whole Art of Midwifery Discovered*. Oxford: Oxford University Press.

Sheils, W.J. (1989) *The English Reformation 1530–1570*. London: Longman Higher Education.

Shiva, Dr. V. (1998) An interview with Dr. Vandana Shiva: 'The deeper you can manipulate living structures the more you can control food and medicine'. St. Louis, Missouri at the First Grassroots Gathering on Biodevastation: Genetic Engineering, on July 18, 1998. Dr. Shiva was the keynote speaker at the conference. The interview was conducted by *In Motion Magazine* publisher Nic Paget-Clarke.

Shy, K.K., Luthy, D.A., Bennett, F.C., Wintfield, M., Larson, E.B., Van Belle, G., Hughes, J.P., Wilson, J.A. and Stenchever, M.A. (1990) 'Effects of Electronic Fetal-heart-rate Monitoring, as compared with Periodic Auscultation, on the Neurologic Development of Premature Infants'. *New England Journal of Medicine*, 322(9).

Sim, J. and Sharp, K. (1998) 'A Critical Appraisal of the Role of Triangulation in Nursing Research'. *International Journal of Nursing Studies*, 35: 23–31.

Sisto, S. and Hillier, D. (1996) 'Advancing and Enhancing Midwifery Practice: Tracking the Impact of a Curriculum Innovation Through a Process of Illuminative Evaluation'. Internal Confederation of Midwives, Conference Proceedings, May 1996.

Skilbeck, M. (1984) *School Based Curriculum Development*. London: Harper and Row.

Skillings, L.N. (1992) 'Perceptions and Feelings of Nurses about Horizontal Violence as an Expression of Oppressed Group Behaviour'. In J.L. Thompson, D.G. Allen and L. Rodrigues-Fisher (eds), *Critique, Resistance and Action: Working Papers in Politics of Nursing*. New York: National League for Nursing Press. pp. 167–185.

Skinner, Q. (1978) *The Foundations of Modern Political Thought*, 2 vols (esp. vol. 2). Cambridge: Cambridge University Press.

Sleep, J., Roberts, J. and Chalmers, I. (1989) 'Care during the second stage of labour'. In I. Chalmers, M. Enkin and Keirse, M.J.N.C. (eds), *Effective care in pregnancy and childbirth*. Oxford: Oxford University Press. pp. 1129–44.

Smith, M.A., Ruffin, M.T. and Green, L.A. (1993) 'The Rational Management of Labor'. *American Family Physician*, 47(6).

Smith, M.C. and Holmes, L.J. (1996) *Listen to Me Good: The Life Story of an Alabama Midwife*. Columbus, Ohio: Ohio State University.

Smith, P.M. (1988) Anti-Piracy News and Copyright Review (Publishers Assn.) June from Blackstone's Guide to the CDPA.

Sontag, S. (1978) *Illness as Metaphor*. New York: Vintage Books.

Sonoma County Peace Press (2000) *Global Resistance of Structural Adjustment Programs*. Sonoma County Peace Press, June/July.

Spivak, G.C. (1976) 'Translator's preface'. In J. Derrida (ed.), *Of Grammatology*. Baltimore, Md.: The Johns Hopkins University Press.

Spring, N. M. and Stern, B. (1998) *Nurse Abuse? Couldn't be!: Intraprofessional Abuse and Violence in the Nursing Workplace*.
http://www.nurseadvocate.org/nurseabuse.html

Stacey, M. and Homans, H. (1978) 'The Sociology of Health and Illness: Its Present State, Future Prospects and Potential for Health Research'. *Sociology*, 12(2): 281–307.

Stanley, L. (ed.) (1990) *Feminist Praxis Research, Theory and Epistemology in Feminist Sociology*. Routledge: London.

Staudt, K. and Col, J-M. (1991) 'Diversity in East Africa: Cultural Pluralism, Public Policy, and the State'. *Women and International Development Annual*, 2: 20–64.

Stone, L. (1986) 'Primary Health Care for Whom? Village Perspectives from Nepal'. *Social Science and Medicine*, 22(3): 293–302.

—— (1992) 'Cultural Influences in Community Participation in Health'. *Social Science and Medicine*, 34(3–4): 409–418.

Strathern, M. (1988) *The Gender of the Gift*. Berkeley, Calif.: University of California Press.

Stringer, E.T. (1996) *Action Research: A Handbook for Practitioners*. London: Sage.

Sullivan, D.A. and Beeman, R. (1983) 'Four Years Experience with Home Birth by Licensed Midwives in Arizona'. *American Journal of Public Health*, 73(6): 641–645.

Susie, D.A. (1988) *In the Way of Our Grandmothers: A Cultural View of Twentieth Century Midwifery in Florida*. Athens, G.A. and London: University of Georgia Press.

Symon, G. and Cassell, C. (eds) (1994) *Qualitative Methods in Organizational Research*. London: Sage.

—— (1998) *Qualitative Methods and Analysis in Organizational Research*. London: Sage.

Symonds, A. and Hunt, S.C. (1996) *The Midwife and Society: Perspectives, Policies and Practice*. London: Macmillan.

Taba, H. (1962) *Curriculum Development: Theory and Practice*. New York: Harcourt, Brace and World.

Tew, M. (1985) 'Safety in Intranatal Care: The Statistics'. In G.N. Marsh (ed.), *Modern Obstetrics in General Practice*. Oxford: Oxford University Press.

—— (1986) 'Do Obstetric Intranatal Interventions Make Birth Safer?' *British Journal of Obstetrics and Gynaecology*, 93: 659–674.

—— (1990) *Safer Childbirth? A Critical History of Maternity Care*. London: Chapman and Hall.

Thomas, B.G. and Cooke, P. (1999) 'Triggering Learning in Midwifery'. *Practising Midwife*, 2(5): 32–34.

Thomas, B.G., Quant, V.M. and Cooke, P. (1998) 'The Development of a Problem-based Curriculum in Midwifery'. *Midwifery*, (14)4: 261–265.

Thomas, J. and Paranjothy, S. (2001) 'National Sentinel Caesarean Section Audit Report'. Royal College of Obstetricians and Gynaecologists Clinical Effectiveness Support Unit. London: RCOG Press.

Thompson, M. (1990) *Cultural Theory*. Boulder, Colo. and Oxford: West View.

—— (1992) 'The dynamics of cultural theory and their implications for the enterprise culture'. In S. Heap and A. Ross (eds), *Understanding the Enterprise Culture: Themes in the Work of Mary Douglas*. Edinburgh: Edinburgh University Press. pp. 182–198.

Titchen, A. (1993) 'Action Research as a Research Strategy: Finding our way through a philosophical and methodological maze'. In *Changing Nursing Practice through Action Research*. Oxford: National Institute for Nursing.

Treicher, P.A. (1990) 'Feminism, Medicine, and the Meaning of Midwifery'. In M. Jacobus, E. Fox Keller and S. Shuttleworth (eds), *Body/Politics: Women and the Discourse of Science*. New York: Routledge. pp. 113–138.

Tritten, J. (1999) 'Freedom'. *Midwifery Today*, 52 (Winter): 1.

Tsing, A. L. (1990) 'Monster Stories: Women Charged with Perinatal Endangerment'. In Faye Ginsberg and Anna Lowenhaupt Tsing (eds), *Uncertain Terms: Negotiating Gender in American Culture*. Boston: Beacon. pp. 282–299.

Turner, V. (1969) *The Ritual Process: Structure and Anti-Structure*. Chicago: Aldine.

—— (1979) 'Betwixt and Between: The Liminal Period in Rites de Passage'. In W. Lessa and E.Z. Vogt (eds), *Reader in Comparative Religion*, (4th edn). New York: Harper & Row.

Tyler, R.W. (1949) *Basic Principles of Curriculum and Instruction*. Chicago: University of Chicago Press.

United Kingdom Central Council For Nursing, Midwifery and Health Visiting (2000) Requirements for pre-registration midwifery programmes. Registrar's Letter 25/2000 SN/JS/JK 18th September. London: UKCC.

United Nations (1974) *New International Economic Order*. United Nations General Assembly.

United Nations Children's Fund (1989) *All for Health: A Resource Book for Facts for Life*. Geneva: UNICEF.

—— (1991) *Draft Master Plan of Operations for the HMG-UNICEF Nepal Programme of Cooperation for the Period 1992–1996*. Kathmandu: UNICEF-Nepal. (United Nations Children's Fund and His Majesty's Government of Nepal).

—— (1996) *Progress of Nations*. Geneva: UNICEF.

United Nations Education and Scientific Cultural Organization (2000) *Best Practice on Indigenous Knowledge Successful Projects Related to Poverty and Social Exclusion*. UNESCO. *http://www.unesco.org/most/bphome.htm#6*

UNHCR News (1999) *Kosovo Crisis Update* Wednesday 8th September. *http://www.unhcr.ch/news/media/kosovo.htm*

United Nations Interim Administration in Kosovo (2000) *Bringing Peace to Kosovo.*
    http://www.un.org/peace/kosovo/pages/kosovo1.htm

Usher, R. (1992) 'Experience in Adult Education: A Postmodern Critique'. *Journal of Philosophy*, 26(2): 212.

US Department of Commerce Economics and Statistics Administration (1995) *Women in the United States: A Profile.* Bureau of Census SB.95–19RV.

US Department of Labor (2001) *20 Leading Occupations of Employed Women 2001 Annual Averages.* US Department of Labor Women's Bureau.
    http://www.dol.gov/wb/wb_pubs/20lead2001.htm

Van Alten, D., Eskes M. and Treffers P.E. (1989) 'Midwifery in the Netherlands; the Wormerveer study: Selection, Mode of Delivery, Perinatal Mortality and Infant Morbidity. *British Journal of Obstetrics and Gynaecology*, 96: 656–662.

Van Binsbergen, W.M.J. (1999) *Virtuality as a Key Concept in the Study of Globalisation: Aspects of the Symbolic Transformation of Contemporary Africa.* Web Book second edition. First published 1997 The Hague: WOTRO Working Paper No. 3.
    http://home.soneraplaza.nl/mw/prive/vabin/gen3/virtuality%20map/virt0.htm

Van der Vlugt T. and Piotrow, P. T. (1974) 'Menstrual Regulation Update'. *Population Report Series* 4: 49–64. Washington, DC: George Washington University Medical Centre.

Van Gennep, A. (1966) *The Rites of Passage.* Chicago, Ill.: University of Chicago Press.

Verber, C.H. (1995) 'International Credentialing of Midwives in Midwifery Today, Inc'. *International Midwife*, 2.
    http://www.midwiferytoday.com/articles/intercred.htm

Verderese, Maria de Lourdes, and Turnbull, Lily M. (1975) *The Traditional Birth Attendant in Maternal and Child Health and Family Planning: A Guide to Her Training and Utilization.* Geneva: World Health Organization.

Vivian, J. (1995) *Adjustment, Globalization and Social Development Seminar Report.* United Nations Research Institute for Social Development. Geneva: Switzerland.
    http://www.unrisd.org/engindex/publ/list/conf/glb1/glb1–03.htm#P156_6653

Vogt, E.Z. (1976) *Tortillas for the Gods: A Symbolic Analysis of Zinacanteco Rituals.* Cambridge, Mass.: Harvard University Press.

Wade, R. (2001) 'Winners and Losers'. *The Economist*, April.

Wallerstein, I. (1974) *The Modern World-System, I: Capitalist Agriculture and the Origins of the European World-Economy in the Sixteenth Century.* New York: Academic Press.

—— (1980) *The Modern World-System, II: Mercantilism and the Consolidation of the European World-Economy, 1600–1750.* New York: Academic Press.

—— (1987) 'World Systems Analysis'. In A. Giddens and J. Turner (eds), *Social Theory Today*. Stanford: Stanford University Press. pp. 309–324.

—— (1989) *The Modern World-System III: The Second Era of Great Expansion of the Capitalist World-Economy, 1730–1840.* New York: Academic Press.

—— (1990a) 'Culture as the Ideological Battleground of the Modern World-System'. *Theory, Culture and Society* 7. London: Sage. pp. 31–55.

—— (1990b) 'Culture is the World-system: A Reply to Boyne'. In M. Featherstone (ed.), *Global Culture: Nationalism, Globalization and Modernity*. London: Sage.

Walsh, J. and Warren, K.S. (1979) 'Selective Primary Health Care: An Interim Strategy for Disease Control in Developing Countries'. *New England Journal of Medicine*, 301(180): 967–974.

Warner, M., Longley, M., Gould, E. and Picek, A. (1998) *Health Care Futures 2010.* London: United Kingdom Central Council for Nurses, Midwives & Health Visitors.

Waters, M. (1995) *Globalization.* London: Routledge.

Weber, M. (1976) *The Protestant Ethic and the Spirit of Capitalism.* London: Allen and Unwin. (First published 1904–5).

Webster's New Collegiate Dictionary (1979) Springfield, Mass.: Merriam.

Wenzel, E. (1997) 'Environment, Development and Health. Ideological Metaphors of Post-traditional Societies?' *Health Education Research,* 12(4): 403–418.

Wertz, R.W. and Wertz, D.C. (1989) *Lying-In: A History of Childbirth in America.* (revised edn). New Haven: Yale University Press.

Wilkinson, R. (2000) *Mind the Gap: Hierarchies, Health and Human Evolution,* London: Weidenfeld & Nicholson.

Williams, R. (1983) 'Concepts of Health: An Analysis of Lay Logic'. *Sociology,* 17(2): 185–205.

Williams, R.M. Jr (1970) *American Society. A Sociological Interpretation.* New York: Knopf.

Winter, R. (1989) *Learning from Experience: Principles and Practice in Action Research.* London: Falmer Press.

Wodak, R. (1995) 'Power, Discourse and Styles of Female Leadership in School Committee Meetings'. In D. Corson (ed.), *Discourse and Power in Educational Organizations.* Cresskill, N.J.: Hampton Press. pp. 31–54.

Women's Global Network for Reproductive Rights (1992) Report of the Maternal Mortality and Morbidity Campaign. Amsterdam.

Wood, G. (1985) 'The Politics of Development Policy Labeling'. *Development and Change,* 16: 348–359.

World Bank (1998) *Social Consequences of the East Asian Financial Crisis.* Washington, D.C.: World Bank.

—— (1999) World Development Indicators 1999. Washington, D.C.: World Bank.

World Health Organization (1975) *Traditional Birth Attendants: A Field Guide to Their Training, Evaluation, and Articulation with Health Services.* Geneva: World Health Organization.

—— (1978) *Primary Health Care: Report of the International Conference on Primary Health Care, Alma-Ata, USSR,* 6–12 September. Jointly sponsored by the World Health Organization and the United Nations Children's Fund. Geneva: World Health Organization.

—— (1985) *Having a Baby in Europe.* Copenhagen: WHO Regional Office for Europe.

—— (1986) *Safe Motherhood.* Geneva: World Health Organization.

—— (1986) Evaluation of the Strategy for Health for All by the Year 2000. Seventh Report on the World Health Situation, Vol 4: South-east asia Region. New Delhi: Regional Office for South-east Asia, World Health Organization.

—— (1988) *Division of Child Health and Development: Improving Child Health.* WHO/CHD 97.12, Geneva: World Health Organization.

—— (1992) *Traditional Birth Attendants: A Joint WHO/UNFPA/UNICEF Statement.* Geneva: World Health Organization.

—— (1992a) *Safe Motherhood Newsletter.* Geneva: World Health Organization.

—— (1992b) *Commission on Health and Environment: Our Planet, Our Health.* Geneva: World Health Organization.

—— (1996) *The World Health Report 1996. Fighting Disease, Fostering Development.* Geneva: World Health Organization.

—— (1996) *Revised 1990 Estimates of Maternal Mortality: A New Approach by WHO and UNICEF.* Geneva: World Health Organization.

—— (1999) *Care in Normal Birth: A Practical Guide. Report of a Technical Working Group WHO/FRH/MSM/96.24* Geneva: World Health Organization, Department of Reproductive Health and Research.

—— (1999) *World Health Report: Making a Difference.* Geneva: World Health Organization.

Worsley, P. (1990) 'Models of the Modern World-System'. In M. Featherstone (ed.) *Global Culture: Nationalism, Globalization and Modernity.* London: Sage.

Young, M. (1971) *Knowledge and Control: New Directions in the Sociology of Education.* London: Collier-Macmillan.

Young, G. and Drife, J. (1992) 'Home or hospital birth?' *Practitioner*, 236(1515): 672–674.

Young G. and Hey, E. (2000) 'Choosing between Home and Hospital Delivery. Home Birth in Britain can be Safe'. *British Medical Journal*, 320(7237): 798.

Zerubavel, E. (1981) *Hidden Rhythms: Schedules and Calendars in Social Life.* Chicago, Ill.: University of Chicago Press.

—— (1985) *The Seven Day Circle.* New York: Free Press.

Index